The Healing Mind

By the same author

The Power of the Mind (with Simon Petherick)

The
Healing Mind

Healing Through Self-hypnosis and Therapeutic Regression

JOE KEETON
with
MONICA O'HARA

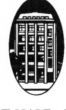

ROBERT HALE · LONDON

© Joe Keeton with Monica O'Hara 1998
First published in Great Britain 1998

ISBN 0 7090 6147 1

Robert Hale Limited
Clerkenwell House
Clerkenwell Green
London EC1R 0HT

2 4 6 8 10 9 7 5 3 1

Typeset in Bembo
by Derek Doyle & Associates, Mold, Flintshire
Printed in Great Britain by
St Edmundsbury Press Limited, Bury St Edmunds
and bound by
WBC Book Manufacturers Limited, Bridgend

Contents

Part Three: When Hypnotherapy can Help

Part Four: Digging Deep into the Mind

This book is dedicated to Sister Gwyneth Poacher, MBE, and her hard-working team of carers and volunteers at the Sandville Self Help Centre who are an inspiration to us all.

Acknowledgements

I should like to express my thanks to all the patients, their families, carers, nurses and doctors who have been kind enough to co-operate in the preparation of this book.

Introduction

In January 1997, I received a spontaneously-written letter which was typical of many sent by patients eager to let me know of their progress. The message contained in this one represented an encouraging start to the New Year.

Cathy Groeger, a college student living in Bournemouth, wrote: 'You may remember I came to see you with my new husband, David, last May? This is just to let you know that we are both feeling much better since then. The eczema patches David had on his legs have almost entirely disappeared and I continue to benefit from what you taught me.'

Cathy's enthusiastic letter continued: 'I find written exams much easier since you helped me. My health is better than it has ever been and improves all the time. I feel wonderful!

'David graduated as a chiropractor in September and is now working at a complementary health centre. I finish my five-year course later this year and I shall keep you informed of our progress.'[1]

The improvements in Cathy's and David's health were due to the fact that, having been taught self-hypnosis in order to re-activate dormant abilities deep inside them, they were practising the technique on a daily basis. While it is true that I had acted as catalyst − as I do in all such cases − their continued health improvements were due entirely to their own efforts.

My entire philosophy is based on the tenet that all cases of *genuine* hypnosis are *self* hypnosis and, on that basis, I focus on teaching patients how to use their own minds to rectify whatever part of the body is malfunctioning. If we regard the brain's internal information system as a sort of computer, it begins to make sense. The conscious mind becomes console and the subconscious (now more commonly known as the unconscious nervous system, or UNS) its processor.

The UNS controls the heartbeat, blood pressure, respiration and all those other bodily functions necessary for our survival. Since millennia animals, then humans, have developed an ability to repel foreign substances, to keep us alive. Our immune system must be capable of continually surveying our internal environment to detect these foreign substances, in order to react to and eliminate them. When the body's defence mechanism breaks down, we become ill. A flawed immune system renders us particularly susceptible to disease. Reactivating the immune system means combining antibodies with antigens to fight off invading substances in the body, thus protecting it from outside influences. The hypnotic method adopted to bring about this phenomenon will be examined presently; but first, we need to look at the connection between our body's defence mechanism and the bank of memories stored in the vaults of our unconscious – in other words, to investigate what really activates the healing mind.

The immune system, as I interpret it, is a set of distant memories of whatever substances the body should produce to fight off those foreign substances automatically eliminated by our long-dead ancestors. It is my contention that these memories need reactivating rather than suppressing. Reactivated memories can vigorously attack malfunctioning cells, whereas synthetic drugs reduce our resistance and therefore provoke the wrong immune response. They therefore potentially place us at risk. Like any other technique this one must be practised regularly, otherwise the ability will be lost. Cathy and David are just two of hundreds to have benefited from learning to use their minds correctly.

Cathy's letter went on to explain that David was now working at a new complementary healthcare centre set up by a group of doctors in Bournemouth; a centre where she too hoped to be employed on completion of her five-year college course. She had found self-hypnosis beneficial in terms of memory recall when dealing with examination papers and was confident that it would help her in a similar way through her finals.

I must make it clear at the outset that I am not a healer, but someone who has an ability to help others heal themselves: a 'persuader' would be my word of choice. While I provide the key to the door connecting the conscious and unconscious parts of the mind, it is up to patients themselves whether they turn that key, unlock the door and access the huge bank of long-lost memories, with all their accompanying potential. Influencing the mind for the benefit of the body is nothing new. On the contrary, it is an age-old ability which animals retain, but which humans have largely lost.

I am more usually known for my work in the field of age regressions, but a personal curiosity in the levels of subconscious activity during sleep led me to investigate just what the UNS *could* do. Working on the premise that it (the UNS) retained the wealth of memories constituting regression, I concluded that it had the capacity to store considerably more data than the conscious. Since the embryonic possibilities were already present within our own minds and bodies, there seemed no logical reason why these memories could not be stimulated into action. Surely these, like any other memories, could be restored to life under the stimulus of hypnosis? If so, that stimulus could bring about dramatic changes in the body's functioning. Tumours could be shrunk. Degenerative diseases of the central nervous system could be stopped in their path; changes instigated could be generalized or specific. I tested the theory and it worked. A whole host of major illnesses and injuries were relieved, many tumour growths inhibited.

I am not claiming that hypnosis can cure cancer, but there have been several instances of tumours going into remission after hypnotic treatment, as we shall see in the following pages. Sceptics might claim that remission merely coincides with the treatment. So be it. The success rate is higher when both are used.

Many patients suffering from cancer visit the Sandville Self Help Centre in South Wales, run by Sister Gwyneth Poacher.[2] I see groups of individuals every month or so. They are suffering from a wide range of physiological and psychological conditions. The Centre offers a variety of treatments alongside hypnosis. These include reflexology, aromatherapy and other methods of healing.

No one is suggesting that the resultant cures are miraculous. They are not brought about by the invocation of any supernatural power, as practitioners are the first to point out. Patients willing and able to undergo complementary therapies alongside conventional methods of treatment have said they find these techniques wholly beneficial. Hypnosis and acupuncture are both strongly recommended for pain relief. Each of these therapies acts by producing endorphins, which are morphine-like substances manufactured in the pituitary gland at the base of the brain. Endorphins help regulate the heart and blood pressure and are believed to be produced under conditions of extreme pain and stress.

Acupuncture involves inserting tiny needles into the patient's skin along what practitioners of this ancient Chinese therapy refer to as meridians, or channels. The purpose of the needles is to unblock the channels in order to restore health.

Insertion of the needles stimulates peripheral nerves, produces pain (apparently of a different nature from the original) then releases endorphins, which act as natural analgesics (painkillers).

That is all very well in its way, but why insert needles into the skin when, by learning self-hypnosis, the same analgesic effect can be achieved? Given that most acupuncturists are scrupulously careful about sterilizing their needles, there may still be a few who are not, with the result that the very slight possibility of infection does exist. No needles of any type are involved in the teaching of self-hypnosis. It is therefore, in my opinion, a much safer option. Under hypnosis we can be taught to produce our own endorphins. The naturally produced variety are, of course, much more powerful than their pharmaceutically manufactured counterparts and they have no side effects.

Animals are so much better than their human companions in terms of dealing with pain. When patients approach me for treatment I always ask if they have a domestic pet. If so, I suggest they study its behaviour when hurt. A cat or dog will yelp momentarily, then its mental processes spring into action to switch off the pain. That is what we should be able to do, and *are* able to do once we have mastered the art of self-hypnosis.

The purpose of this book, therefore, is to concentrate on the mind's abilities to heal. The pity of it is that, in this so-called Age of Enlightenment as we approach the new millennium, so many people are still totally unaware of the great potential for healing right there inside their own heads.

Note

1. Cathy did keep me informed: updated case histories of her husband and herself are included in Chapter 14.

2. The Sandville Self Help Centre is a registered charity (number 517 889). It is based at Sandville Court, Ton Kenfig, mid Glamorgan, CF33 4PT. Telephone: 01656 743344.

PART ONE
Ancestral Survivors

1 Origins

Sit in front of a computer. Start using the keyboard and watch the message appear on the screen. Generally speaking, information can be retrieved from the storage media at any given time for examination and re-use.

We know the program has been fed into the equipment's memory but we also know that we can only retrieve it if we have learned the correct method of doing so. Otherwise how could we be expected to know that bringing up the program involved inserting the disk, using the keyboard and moving the cursor or mouse to the required spot?

One does not need to be computer-literate to be able to operate equipment at its most basic level. As with a television set, the average individual has no idea how images appear on the screen. Our only concern is that on pressing the relevant keys or buttons and making any other necessary moves these images should appear. If they fail to do so, we call in the experts.

Man's internal computer
A similar situation occurs with the mind. The average individual has no idea how the mind works. It is a matter of no concern unless its function is less than efficient.

The language of computers is complex and not easily understood by non-experts. Like any other language, it has its own vocabulary, but the only words which might concern us here are *disks*, *stored data*, *memory banks* and *errors in the code*.

Throughout our lives data is being fed into and stored by the computer of our mind. From the 'keyboard' of our consciousness, all sorts of programs, images and memories move on to our unconscious memory banks.

Some of the information is retained in the conscious but most of it passes into the unconscious. This is where we differ dramatically from the computer. While even the most powerful computer has a limit to the amount of data it can store, our vastly superior memory banks have the ability to retain everything we have ever seen, read, been told or experienced throughout our lives.

Because nothing is ever deleted from the filing system of our mind, theoretically we should be able to retrieve any of this information once we know how. The correction of any errors in the program should then be possible.

When it comes to our state of health, the most important information in the computer of the mind is the set of memories forming the immune system, as already indicated in the introductory notes. The most damage caused to this set of memories comes from man-made drugs, both the prescribed variety and those purchased over the counter.

Therein lies the crux of the problem. We must be taught which keys to press in order to access the data for those errors to be corrected. *The important issue at stake is that all the information fed in over the years is contained in our memory bank, but remains there unless we know how to access it.* Once the data has been stored, any incorrectly coded programs must be altered in order to restore us to health.

It is my contention that only by means of deep hypnosis can these faulty programs be retrieved and the information corrected. I see the conscious as the information gatherer, thinker, reasoner and the unconscious as the processor of the information gathered.

The evidence coming through strongly from my case histories suggests that, although conscious and unconscious minds can operate independently, reasoning and thought have no place in the unconscious mind. The conscious simply reacts to the programs fed into it over the years, its chief function being to protect life and balance.

With due respect to my colleagues in psychotherapy, I believe their methods invariably fail because of their inability to access those deep-rooted memories. The notion that patients can talk through their problems is perfectly logical if the patients know what they are, but in my experience the most serious problems arise from the presence in the mind of bad memories of which the unconscious mind has buried away from the conscious.

Unconscious mechanisms

The unconscious nervous system (or UNS) is able to react individually from the conscious and it is an established fact – even in traditional medicine – that the unconscious frequently refuses to allow the conscious to remember events which it (the UNS) considers too dangerous for everyday recall. But memories can be distorted. Events which would create terror in the mind of a small child would be dismissed out of hand by an adult.

For example, I find that the memories of many grown men and women are blocked off on their first day at school: understandably, one might think; it is a time of great stress in a young life. Not every five-year-old can cope with being taken away from mother and home for the first time. To be plunged into a frequently overcrowded reception class is bad enough, but having to mix with so many strange children and adults must be infinitely worse; particularly for those inclined to be shy or timid.

Some mental blocks originating from a patient's first day at school have been brought on by more specific difficulties. They can relate to not having the correct uniform, being called names by the school bully, or being teased over an inability to button a blazer. One college lecturer's memories had been blocked because, being unsure where the lavatory was, he had accidentally wet himself in class.

A particularly intriguing case was that of a middle-aged housewife, also regressed to the age of five. Quivering with fear, she was back in her convent preparatory school having her first encounter with nuns. Curiously, it was not the sight of her teachers' long black habits that created panic in the formative young mind, but the fact that the nuns were wearing lace-up shoes of the type associated with police officers. Why the child should have been frightened of the police was quite a different matter and resulted in further regressive therapy, which ultimately involved most members of her family.

The point I am making is that once the lecturer's and the housewife's memories were led back to the day in question and, as adults, they were able to *re-live* (rather than simply remember) the events, their minds accepted that there was no longer anything to fear.

Over and over again I find that the act of bringing these traumas into the open reveals them for what they truly are, thus rendering them harmless to the system. While it is natural for a five-year-old to be frightened on a first day at school, it is not natural for an adult to continue regarding these memories as dangerous twenty years on. The adult's unconscious mind needs convincing that the events, albeit unpleasant at the time, are no longer cause for concern.

The invisible enemy

The sad fact about stress is that we do not even realize we are suffering from it until we exceed our tolerance level. To put it another way, only when something goes snap does the violinist or tennis player realize how taut the fractured string must have been. Unless and until we know the cause of our difficulties we cannot battle with it. Matters must be brought into the light in order for patient and therapist to tackle them.

Otherwise, we are fighting an invisible enemy.

The purpose of regressive hypnotherapy is to enable patients to bring out unknown, unsuspected, aspects of themselves so that they can be dealt with in a responsible manner. Without meaning to harp on about psychotherapists, I imagine it now becomes clear why I take these practitioners to task over the notion that talking through patients' problems at a conscious level can achieve results. Without accessing the unconscious to determine the exact nature of what is wrong, how can the difficulties be resolved?

Medical experts acknowledge that as many as seventy-five per cent of today's illnesses are of what they describe as 'unknown aetiology'. Aetiology is medico-speak for the cause of a disease, which doctors may attribute to genetic, hereditary or environmental factors or, in some cases, exposure to infection. What it boils down to is that they really have no idea what has gone wrong. Again, without knowing the cause of an illness, how can they possibly treat it? This is particularly applicable in cases of chronic depression. Not so long ago, it was common practice for general practitioners to prescribe tranquillizers to dull the senses of, and hopefully diminish the trauma for, their depressed patients.

Although these drugs are still being prescribed, doctors are beginning to seek out alternatives. Quite apart from the obvious dangers of tranquillizer-addiction, patients dependent on these drugs become even more depressed and the more tablets they swallow the more their problems are compounded.

Pill-popping puts matters into the shade. It produces shadows without substance and substance cannot be fought with shadows. As already explained, the substance needs bringing into the light for its reality to be confronted. The beneficial effects of reprogramming the mind by means of regressive hypnotherapy are many and will be examined in more detail presently. All we need to know at this stage is that a variety of programs (correct and otherwise) are fed into the mind in childhood, adolescence and throughout our growing years. In due course, they slip from our conscious memory into the storage vaults of our unconscious. The conscious, because of its overloaded 'disk', cannot retain all of this data.

Yet the unconscious, believing it to be unwise for the conscious to remember anything it considers dangerous, shuts those memories away in its vaults, blissfully unaware of the insidious effect on the system. It builds a symbolic wall between itself and the conscious.

Blocking off bad memories might seem like a good idea at the time, but in the long term, it proves quite the reverse. Unless we can demolish that wall and gain access to the storage vaults, nothing but trouble will result. Unless bad memories are released, all sorts of mental and bodily ills are liable to manifest themselves.

The successful treatment of these ailments is what this book is about. Regression, as anyone who has read *The Power of the Mind*[1] will know, is the technique whereby people are induced into a very deep state of hypnosis and their memories directed back as far as those people are willing or able to go.

Mental blocks

If there are no stumbling-blocks on the way, the memories can race back through the years to the participant's birth, and beyond. Stumbling-blocks, however, frequently crop up and must be removed. Where I differ from others who practise regressive hypnotherapy is that, instead of allowing the memories to hurtle back like brakeless vehicles shooting into reverse, I ask the 'driver' to make frequent, unscheduled, stops on that sloping hill downward, to ensure that they are still in control of their vehicle and that their route is clear. What vehicle can go speeding over a fallen tree, or past a jackknifed lorry? Such obstacles need removing before the journey can be resumed.

Road-blocks – whatever their cause – impede a journey. Mental blocks do likewise. Repressed memories must be brought to the fore and dealt with therapeutically; it is simply not possible to progress until these obstacles have been removed. That is why I stop the memories at various stages in the regressed individual's life. I need to ensure that they can retrieve the events of that time before proceeding further and I make a particular point of using the word 'relive' rather than 'remember'.

This is very important because if, in their state of unconscious recall, people use the past tense, then some of the wall blocking the memory pathway from unconscious to conscious is still there, preventing true regression. Nor does it automatically follow that, even if relating their experiences in the present tense, they are actually experiencing them. If the words are being uttered in a bland, emotionless fashion and the trauma is absent the block is still there. Removing it is crucial for the maintenance of health.

Having acknowledged that our memories are storage vaults for a vast array of experiences, thoughts and ideas and that the most dramatic of these must be brought to the fore and relived, my words invariably include instructions to bring back all the memories, however harrowing that experience might be.

Only when the voice of the person being regressed assumes a younger tone, speaks in the present tense, and the cries are of anguish or anger, is the mental wall demolished. It means that we can unlock the door of the vault and extract all the information we need from the carefully stored files.

Having retrieved the necessary data, we can continue our route backwards; pressing on through earlier times, still stopping, still checking, until every memory pathway is crystal clear. With this in mind, when I am conducting regressions, I am always careful to implant safeguards so that patients suffer no after-effects. Arousing 'regressees' from their hypnotised state, I invariably tell them: 'When you come back, you will feel no pain. Leave behind anything wrong with your mind or body. Come back only with the memories.' The instruction 'You will feel no pain' is mandatory.

When memories are clear and an interesting character emerges from pre-birth experiences, that is a bonus. But, as far as I am concerned, it is not the main object of the exercise. I believe my *raison d'être* is to help people benefit from hypnosis.

That is one reason why I specialise in teaching self-treatment; the other reason is that, among the many other benefits, it avoids emotional dependency. Apart from those patients suffering from long term, intractable conditions, after that initial session of hypnotherapy, patients are expected to treat themselves. The presence of blocks results in stress and stress is not good for us. It is at the root of so many illnesses and is so widespread today that no-one could even hazard a guess as to how many people suffer from its effects. It has been known to produce, or emphasise a host of physical signs and symptoms, even if psychosomatic factors are not always seen to be present. Psoriasis is a case in point.

This is a skin condition characterized by blotchy red patches which, if untreated, itch and flake off in a most embarrassing manner. The disease at its worst can mean associated, painful arthritis and psoriatics know only too well that even after complete disappearance the rash can recur at any time. Of all dermatological conditions, widespread resistant psoriasis is one of the most distressing for the sufferer, and one of the most difficult for doctors to treat. Yet, psoriasis responds readily to hypnosis. So too does acne, a skin condition which in its own way is every bit as unsightly and distressing.

Characterized by angry red blemishes on the face, acne is usually at its most acute in teenagers when examinations are imminent. Though not by any means confined to students, the condition *is* frequently seen among intelligent school-leavers and undergraduates. It is directly related to stress.

Aware of the importance of good results, its young sufferers tend to freeze up and not gain the expected grades, thus compromising their career prospects. With access to the memory bank of the unconscious, an examinee can draw upon any of his or her resources. All the information gleaned from reading or attending class or lectures is there for the taking. Acquiring this ability removes stress-related examination nerves. When the stress goes so does the acne, or whatever other undesirable condition has been manifesting itself in the sufferer.

Most of us understand how hypnosis can be utilized for the treatment of emotional and psychological disorders, what is less easy to understand is how it can relieve physical conditions.

Yet a variety of other skin complaints respond readily to hypnosis. Blood conditions and the various forms of arthritis have also been successfully treated in this way.

Philippa was a medical student, suffering from systemic lupus erythematosus (usually known simply as lupus, or SLE). Systemic conditions are so called because they can involve virtually every part of the body: heart, lungs, kidneys, liver, joints, tendons, even neurological function.

For an attractive young woman like Philippa, the facial manifestations of SLE are particularly distressing. Redness beneath the eyes and across the nose produces the characteristic wolf-like appearance (*lupus* being Latin for wolf), while the word 'erythematosus' relates to the progression of the skin rash.

SLE is sometimes treated with steroids, as indeed are many other chronic conditions such as asthma, bronchitis and rheumatoid arthritis. The unpleasant side-effects of steroids can include peptic ulcers, gastro-intestinal bleeding, high blood pressure, diabetes, anaemia, hair loss and mental confusion. Some have been known actually to cause tumours.

When hypnotherapy is routinely given in addition to conventional therapy (certainly never instead of it), the mind can be instructed to eliminate any unpleasant or dangerous reactions to manufactured drugs. Some drugs developed to treat the various forms of cancer, for example, can have very unpleasant side effects, such as pain, vomiting, skin discoloration and hair loss. More significantly, the drug regime need not even be an aggressive form of chemotherapy; every time any form of medication is introduced into our bodies it suppresses our own internal defences. Using self-hypnosis to help the mind achieve its healing potential has been found to be a much safer option because there are no side effects.

Deep hypnosis is a potent means of healing.

Reaching the control centre

By means of hypnosis it is possible to reach into the control centre of the mind, where the key connecting conscious and unconscious is located. Once I am satisfied that the patient about to undergo hypnosis understands what is happening and provided I have the patient's complete trust and co-operation, I proceed to ease him or her gently into the deepest possible level of hypnosis. Then, communicating directly with the UNS, I find that the 'computer' will respond like any other.

Instructions are given for the body's defences to liven up cellular and biochemical interactions and to rectify malformations. The conscious mind is still aware of what is happening but cannot interfere. However, as a safety precaution I do insist that if my patient experiences even the slightest objection to anything being said or done the UNS will hand back control to the conscious immediately.

Philippa consulted me once only. During that session I hypnotized her and implanted the suggestion in her UNS that she should set about mobilizing whatever processes were necessary to relieve her condition and bring about a generalized improvement in her health.

There is never any question of the hypnotist taking control and, to eliminate the possibility of emotional dependency, I always insist that before leaving my clinic patients put the self-hypnotic technique to the test. They must prove their ability to achieve the necessary level unaided. Having succeeded, they are capable of using their own internal computer to its full capacity. I cannot overemphasize the importance of helping people to help themselves.

Satisfied that Philippa was capable of self-hypnosis as taught, I advised her to make her newly acquired skill a routine daily habit. She did and, according to reports, is faring very well. During her most recent telephone call to me she said her doctor had gradually weaned her off all medication '. . . and my general health is A1'. Hypnosis, she assures me, has been a terrific help, not only for herself but as a potential form of treatment for her own patients, once she gains her medical degree.

Philippa's case history redresses the balance for that of another SLE patient, who must remain anonymous. This second patient did learn self-hypnosis, practised it for a short time, then suddenly began to doubt her new-found ability. Her self-treatment became spasmodic until it ceased altogether. As the symptoms of her condition began to trouble her again she rejected self-hypnosis entirely and turned to other forms of treatment, none of which produced the desired result.

'One of these days, I'll try hypnosis again,' she has promised herself.

I hate to disillusion the poor woman but frankly, there would not be much point in consulting *me* again. I could only repeat the previous procedure, with a result similar to before. I could do no more than encourage her, as I did last time, to practise on a daily basis. If she refuses to do so then I cannot help her. It is not my abilities as a hypnotherapist which this woman is doubting, but those of her own mind. And she herself is the only person who can resolve that problem.

The case of Hazel, a young woman seriously injured in a road traffic accident, has a happier outcome. Hazel was given hypnotherapy to relieve the pain in her right arm, which had been badly fractured. She subsequently found that not only could she control the pain, but movement in the arm was increased. How did she manage this? Like all my patients, Hazel was taught self-hypnosis, originally to gain access to that all-important UNS. Having learned the technique, she continued to practise on a regular basis, finding it an ideal way to cope with most of her health problems at source.

Warts, which seem to appear for no specific reason, can disappear equally mysteriously; on the other hand they can be particularly persistent and defy all methods of cure. The same phenomenon appears to apply to a variety of other tumours, malignant and benign, which after treatment by hypnosis are liable to vanish without any tissue-scarring, sometimes without trace. However, very few doctors will admit that growths will respond to anything other than chemotherapy, radiotherapy or surgical excision.

Cellular messages

Fundamentally, I believe unwelcome bodily manifestations appear because of incorrect messages being beamed out from the brain. We know that the brain's messengers keep instructing the body's cells about what is going on inside us. We also know that if an incorrect instruction is conveyed, or if the instruction is correct but the cells misinterpret its meaning, the body begins to malfunction.

How this comes about is by means of a complicated biochemical procedure, the explanation of which can be found in many readily available text books by those who wish to pursue the matter.

A simple way of spelling it out to the non-scientist might be to think in terms of televised images. Most of us appreciate that if the receiver of our TV set goes out of action the screen will go blank.

Nor should we have difficulty in accepting that if a transmitter goes awry it will cut off the picture, not just on our set but on every set in the area.

As thinkers, we each have our own individual interpretations and some might hold that my personal views are over-simplified, but I believe they are at least worthy of consideration. As I understand it, what happens in our bodies is that if a single cell misinterprets the message being conveyed by the brain, any resultant malignancy is likely to be localized; whereas, if the entire message beaming out from the brain is incorrect the disease, should it occur, is likely to be widespread.

The computer comparison with our mental abilities has already been explored. Let us now approach the subject from a different angle.

Consider the concept of the party-goer who has entered a noisy room with his tape recorder. Imagine he has left the machine at the side of his chair, accidentally switched on. Having forgotten all about it he proceeds to enjoy the festivities. The party becomes noisier but our merrymaker manages to converse relatively normally and also to hear every word spoken directly to him. He picks up all the personal compliments, the odd scandal, the juicy bits of gossip; if someone mentions his name across the proverbial crowded room he automatically turns to see who has spoken.

At the end of the evening the party-goer suddenly remembers the machine on which he intended recording a spot of karaoke and apologizes to his friends for the fact that he never got around to it. It is only on arrival back home that he realizes the record button had been switched on all evening, its full tape having already run back. So he probably *did* manage to record the karaoke after all.

Pressing the play button, he listens out for the hilarious Elvis and Spice Girls interpretations. Instead, out flows an incomprehensible mixture of song and speech: a gabble of distorted sounds. More surprising still, in the general mêlée the man's own voice is indistinguishable from the others. The conscious memory, like the party-goer at the time of the actual event, notes only what is relevant to the moment and ignores all else. The unconscious memory, like the tape recorder, takes absolutely everything on board (much of it of no consequence). If our man or any of his friends want to identify or extract individual voices from the tape it will be necessary to call upon the services of someone experienced in that type of work.

In like manner, if we are to extract specific information from the volume of matter in the UNS we need the assistance of someone with that particular type of expertise – which is where I come in!

Helping patients gain access to the deepest regions of their mind is the prime focus of my work.

Legacy of our primitive ancestors

Man is the product of strong, primitive ancestors who survived only because they *were* strong – and fit. The fact that they passed on their genetic superiority to their offspring raises many questions. *Why* did they survive, where are we – the twentieth-century sophisticates – going wrong, and has civilization somehow rendered us effete?

The UNS, as already mentioned, is an assorted collection of loves, hates, fears and goodness knows what else. It is active from the moment of conception; and has been, right back to the beginning of time. There is no longer any doubt that data, from infancy and earlier, are filed away in our computer's memory and can, as we have seen, be recalled for re-use, then be filed away again. Or they can be left *in situ* and ignored.

Babies are born with inbuilt reflexes which enable them to cry, to search for their mother's nipple and to suck. During the first few weeks and months of their life they begin to recognize other textures, smells, sounds and sensations.

Therefore, accepting that everything is being programmed in their young minds, we know that all those new experiences are storing up in their brains. As the babies become children, adolescents, adults, some memories from their ever-increasing collection can be revived at will; others need a little help; which brings us back to regressive hypnosis (a phenomenon I tend to attribute to inherited memory).

Without turning this into a biology lesson, all I would say here is that we do know that the cell from the mother contains memories of what it must do to manufacture the child, and so on into future generations. We know, too, that one of those sets of memories makes up the immune system. To return to the computer analogy, the idea of the human mind being described as a warehouse stocked full of wisdom makes sense. Man has the capacity to program his own computer; all he needs is someone to show him how.

The inability of the unconscious to realize that circumstances can alter dangerous emotional events into harmless episodes has already been demonstrated. So too has the explanation of why it causes phobias and depressions to make the conscious mind avoid certain situations or events.

In the introductory notes I described the immune system as a set of memories of what the body should produce to counteract the effects of viruses and germs. While theoretically we are still capable of producing the antibodies necessary to protect us, in practical terms the effect of mutated viruses has destroyed – or at least weakened – that protection in most of us.

Buried memories of the immune system need reactivating if we are not to forget completely how to heal ourselves in the way our ancestors did. We must reactivate dormant abilities in the same way that a physiotherapist reactivates the limbs of patients after lengthy periods of immobility. Otherwise the mind, or the limbs, become atrophied.

No one is claiming that hypnosis is a panacea for all ills, but it can be a powerful therapeutic tool. Using regression to revive dormant memories and brain cells, I give many patients access to their own unconscious mind in order to treat, with some considerable success, allergies, phobias, depressions and innumerable psychological and physiological disorders.

This chapter began by focusing on the similarities between the computer and the human mind, so I should like to end along the same lines by stating that, despite the similarities, they differ in two fundamental ways.

Firstly, the complexities of the computer are as nothing compared with those of the human mind. The essential difference is that while the storage memory on the computer can fill up, the capacity of the human version is infinite. Also, the unconscious is well able to operate for itself, but no man-made machine – however sophisticated – could be given that ability. Never, in a million years of computer processing, could man create or clone the intricacies of the human mind . . . or its remarkable power for healing.

Note
1 Keeton, Joe with Simon Petherick, *The Power of the Mind* (Robert Hale 1989).

2   Self-hypnosis

Method

'I am now going to relax for ten minutes and when I come back each part of my body will be growing only its own kind of cell, each part of my body destroying any of the wrong kind of cell already grown.'

Patients who have already proved themselves capable of entering hypnosis give instructions such as these to their own unconscious mind. *En route* to the hypnotic state, they read the words from a specially prepared card, then they count from one to ten to ease themselves into the required depth for self-treatment. The speed of response varies from one individual to another, just as it does when patients are being anaesthetized for surgical procedures in a hospital theatre. In some cases, as the conscious hands over to the UNS, patients do not even manage to reach as far as ten because they are already completely relaxed.

My clinics at home, in London and in South Wales, are all well stocked with 'customized' cards, not just for new patients, but for anyone in need of a *booster*. When setting out to see groups of patients I like to ensure that my briefcase contains a plentiful supply of cards. They accompany me to lectures and group meetings wherever I go, be they regular bases in the British Isles or occasional seminars and workshops and lecture tours further afield. Some provide instructions regarding relaxation and sleep. Others concentrate on stress-removal. Note the word *removal* rather than *management*, which has become something of a buzz word in contemporary society.

When I am approached by patients known to be already suffering from cancer – or, indeed, any other definitively diagnosed

34

condition – the cards relay a different message to their unconscious mind. This time the instructions are to ensure that none of the prescribed medications will suppress or interfere with the immune system, or cause any dangerous side effects. Others might need to instruct their UNS to replace with healthy living cells any already adversely affected by surgical or medical intervention.

Before we part company I like to satisfy myself that patients understand what they are being asked to do and that they can actually do it. They are given the relevant printed cards and advised to read them daily in order to induce themselves into hypnosis. I recommend this as a daily practice because of the previously explained similarity between the workings of the human mind and the everyday computer. We know that if a computer programmer makes even a tiny error in the instruction being fed to his machine, the machine will not recognize the instruction and will fail to respond. Feed in just one inaccurate word or phrase to the brain during hypnosis and it will fail in like manner. Memorizing the necessary words is fine if the patient gets them exactly right, but not everyone does.

Those for whom the daily practice of self-hypnosis as taught becomes as much a habit as cleaning the teeth or setting off to work report a marked improvement in their condition. When the treatment succeeds there are undoubted health benefits. When it fails it is usually because the technique is no longer being practised. This latter group of patients eventually drift back to the way they were before seeking treatment, as demonstrated by the student suffering from SLE, whose story was related in the previous chapter.

In the third category are those who contact me months, or even years, after their initial consultation. When they say their problem has returned and I question them about whether they are still practising the technique, they insist that they are, then confess to having also taken up meditation, yoga, or some other form of mind–body control.

Those people are attempting to make their conscious mind do something for which it is not designed: namely, to take over one of the duties of the unconscious. As a result they cause inner confusion. It is hardly surprising that messages being transmitted from the UNS are equally confused.

Stress-management is big business among the new breeds of psychologists, sociologists and counsellors. Suddenly, it is trendy, with everyone from rising young executives to their stressed-out grandmothers clamouring to have a go. While some of these facilities are obtainable under the National Health Service others are not and vast sums of money are being paid out by anxious and worried people in search of some meaning to their lives. The search has become quite an obsession in some quarters. While there is no doubt that stress is at the root of many ills in our society today, I do not altogether accept that every psychologist has the knowledge or experience to cope with it. Laudable though their efforts to put the world to rights may be, the theory behind the practice is questionable.

Although I do sometimes suggest to people who have not succeeded in entering hypnosis to ask their GP for referral to a *behavioural* psychologist, as I see it society is no more responsible for producing disease than it is for producing criminals. It is such a shame that today's doctors have so many demands on their time, preventing them from devoting more of their energy and expertise to sufferers of stress. Overcrowded surgeries and waiting-rooms are not exactly conducive to their treatment of patients suffering from anxiety neurosis.

Those doctors with whom I have discussed the matter admit they do not like having to reach for the prescription pad, but believe mild tranquillizers have a calming effect by preventing such patients from overreacting, by helping them cope. They know full well that tablets are not the long-term answer. No doctor wants to condemn patients to permanent residence in what journalists colourfully describe as Valium Valley or Prozac Parade. I am not challenging the integrity of doctors. What saddens me is the fact that they are too hard-pressed to devote more than a few minutes to each individual entering their surgeries and health centres.

Liaising with doctors
Doctors who refer patients to me – as they do, increasingly –

acknowledge the need for other forms of treatment alongside their own, or even, when conventional therapy fails, instead of it. That, however, is a decision only they can make. In all other circumstances I believe hypnotherapy should be used in conjunction with conventional techniques. It would be both arrogant and irresponsible of me to suggest otherwise.

Of course, traditional medicine has its place as a major part in the healing process and doctors are always welcome to attend my clinics, either with or without their patients.

Few among us would attach more importance to the alleviation of symptoms than the search for a cure, to the concentration on the disease rather than on the person suffering from it.

There is much to be said for getting back to basics. With a properly functioning immune system it is possible to fight virtually anything without having to resort to outside influences. I do firmly believe that hypnosis can work alongside conventional medicine to prevent dependence on drugs (however mild) with their unpredictable side effects. The idea behind teaching patients to treat themselves is to help them gain more from their lives and to prevent problems from impinging on their day-to-day activities. Hypnosis, therefore, can be a valuable therapeutic tool and should not be used as a stage act or parlour game. The workings of the human mind should never be associated with fun practices.

Stage performers

Questions are sometimes raised about the hypnotic state of those who participate in stage shows. My own opinion is that if the participants were truly deep into hypnosis they would not comply with the daft instructions being given for the entertainment of the audience. The UNS is incapable of imagination or pretence; these properties are the exclusive preserve of the conscious mind.

The stage hypnotist, aiming at entertainment, does not use the gentle, relaxed approach of the therapist, but with typical showmanship tries to get large numbers of people into a state of 'light trance' as quickly as possible. The stage performer makes extensive use of the post-hypnotic signal and of positive and negative hallucinations to make people act foolishly.

He might suggest, for example, that his subject is being chased around the stage by someone or something unseen, which suggestion, when acted upon by the person under hypnosis, is all very entertaining for the audience, but the operator seldom troubles to determine beforehand whether those taking part in his act suffer from any specific fears or phobias. Should the man being chased already have a persecution complex, being told to behave in this way could do untold damage to his mind. Similarly, someone instructed to imagine that he was walking on a tightope could be seriously harmed if, unknown to the hypnotist, he was a sufferer of vertigo.

To create a negative hallucination it is suggested that the man or woman taking part in the act will not see something which is actually there. Although in many instances those who volunteer to participate in stage experiments have such outgoing personalities that they may actually seek to be made to look foolish, there are occasions when members of the audience may be drawn in unwittingly. The unethical type of stage hypnotist may get those people to make fools of themselves once but, unless they are extreme extroverts, they will not do it again, which is of no real consequence to the hypnotist as he is unlikely to see them again.

It is, however, only fair to point out that the top-flight stage hypnotists do have their own code of ethics: it is not the purpose of this book to point any finger of accusation in the direction of entertainers, but merely to illustrate the essential differences between therapists and stage performers.

The theatrical performer may, for example, instruct those participating in his act that the way to count is 'one, two, three, four, five, six, eight, nine, ten' and on being aroused from hypnosis, they will obligingly omit the seven as suggested. This will set up a state of confusion in the mind, whereby they are left wondering why the habit of a lifetime should suddenly be wrong, but no harm is caused if they are put back under hypnosis and told it was a trick and that they can now count correctly.

In the eyes of the general public, those co-operating with the stage hypnotist appear to lose human dignity and their actions throw into disrepute the whole concept of hypnosis; this public image of the operator causes fear and reluctance to undergo hypnosis on the part of people who could very well benefit from hypnotherapy.

Loss of control

What about the accusation relating to so-called loss of control: handing the mind over to someone else, and all the other arguments put forward by people who admit that they know nothing about hypnosis? The simple answer is that this is not what happens. As already pointed out, the only *person* to whom anyone is handing over is in their own unconscious mind. When my voice hits the sleep rhythm inside the patient's head it unlocks the key of the door leading into it. That is all. The rest is up to the individual concerned.

Once the conscious part of the mind has allowed the unconscious to take over and the direct link between the two has been established, vital processes can be motivated. When inducing patients into deep hypnosis I direct their attention to those parts of the body which are not functioning efficiently. Because primitive defence mechanisms are being aroused, when I set about mobilizing these innate resources patients undergoing hypnosis often say they feel energy pulsing through the system. They tell me it manifests itself in a warmth or a tingling which is strongest in whichever part of the body needs most attention. Thus does the link between conscious and unconscious parts of the mind enable people to reawaken long dormant abilities, to improve mental and physical capacities.

Palliative measures are fine in themselves, but the ideal solution is to reach the root of the problem and dispose of it. In most cases where patients have been trained to treat themselves the cycle of problem-dependence-more-problems-more-dependence is broken. The confidence gained from realizing that they are in control of their own situation is half-way to a cure. Again, there are limitations and the first lesson the sufferer must learn is how to distinguish between the actual physical condition and the mental state associated with it.

A fractured limb is purely physical and hypnosis can do nothing to heal the bone; the pain from the injury is mental and can be removed by this particular form of mind-training, but only on a temporary basis and for initial pain-relief. While the patient is in a state of self-hypnosis, I emphasize repeatedly the importance of instructing one's own unconscious mind to correct any bodily malfunctions.

Knowing that pain is sometimes necessary to diagnose an illness, critics of self-induced hypnosis argue that suppressing the pain may lead the sufferer into believing the condition no longer needs attention and that treatment that covers or diminishes pain could make an illness difficult to diagnose or mask its symptoms altogether.

Aware of the danger, I explain to all those seeking hypnosis for therapeutic purposes that pain is like an alarm clock which, having awakened the sufferer to danger, can be switched off until the necessary action is taken. The fractured bone still needs setting, the persistent toothache always needs investigation. The dangers of using self-hypnosis to cover up bodily malfunction or injury are obvious. In passing, I wonder if those people who condemn self-hypnosis for the temporary relief of pain also condemn aspirin and other analgesics readily available without a doctor's prescription: and whether they stop to consider those all-important side-effects.

Another argument put forward by the uninitiated: those who feel they do not wish to be dependent on another person speak of the importance of upholding the privacy of the intellect and retaining their individuality. This is nonsense; there is no question of one person 'imposing his will' on another. All I do is open up the link between conscious and unconscious minds, to teach people how to use an extra part of their own brain, the mechanics of which have already been explained.

What hypnosis is

But what exactly is hypnosis?

The dictionary definition is usually given as 'a state resembling sleep' which in a very superficial way is partly correct, even if only inasmuch as the sleeper and the person under hypnosis both generally have their eyes closed and are in most circumstances deeply relaxed. But there the similarities end because, in the hypnotic state, the person concerned must be fully aware of the surroundings in order to hear the operator's voice and respond to directives.

People being hypnotized for therapeutic purposes are fully alert all the time. Indeed, they experience a *heightened* sense of awareness, both of the operator and of the outside noises and circumstances, mainly because during the initial relaxation process the instructions always include advice to be fully aware, and to cancel if anything dangerous or objectionable threatens. As we shall see in chapter five, one woman did bring herself out of hypnosis when an innocently mentioned word was found to have connotations of which I was unaware at the time.

Having established the connection, and eliminated the problem, she proceeded to re-enter hypnosis, this time without difficulty.

During hypnosis the senses seem sharpened and more acute in some way; even if the power over movement is somewhat reduced those who have been hypnotized describe its state as a strange yet pleasant sensation, both relaxing and stimulating. Typical are the observations of a couple of journalists who came to interview me on separate occasions, each wanting to experience hypnosis for themselves.

The first, a young man, responded to the induction process very quickly and subsequently wrote: 'Joe's lilting voice soon began to affect me. My vision began to blur, my hearing sharpened and I experienced a sensation rather like that of being under gas in the dentist's, but without the bad taste in my mouth.'[1] This writer went on to say that he could hear everything being said, but felt like 'a mind trapped inside a body'.

The second, a prizewinning feature writer on our local evening newspaper, wrote: 'He persuades you into a generally more relaxed state of mind before he starts on the steady, lulling voice tactics which eventually lure you over the alertness borderline and into semi-consciousness . . . imperceptibly, the intellectual need to fight the hypnosis seemed to be ebbing away.' This young woman went on to describe how my voice soon began to 'swivel away from source' and relocate itself inside her own head.[2]

The inducing of patients into hypnosis should involve no instruments, no swinging clocks or beaming lights. There should be no instructions to stare at anything which has a frequency that could be reproduced under different circumstances, such as windscreen wipers or flickering disco lights.

Inbuilt safeguards

It is vitally important to eliminate the possibility of car drivers accidentally re-entering hypnosis as attention becomes fixed on windscreen wipers swinging to and fro. As a further precaution, I invariably stress many times over that anyone being taught self-hypnosis by me will never fall asleep at the wheel of a car, the controls of an aeroplane, or whatever mode of transport they happen to use on a regular basis.

After a few moments the breathing becomes slower, deeper and more regular. Only when the patient is sufficiently deeply hypnotized can any attempt be made to give practical help for the conditions from which he or she might be suffering. Some conditions, being of nervous origin – speech defects, tension headaches, fingernail biting, for example – are notoriously intractable to normal medical methods.

As a general rule, I have found that conditions which can be successfully treated by hypnosis tend to fall into several distinct areas: the psychological with no obvious physical symptoms such as fears, phobias and depressions, and the psychological problems which manifest themselves with physical symptoms, such as migraine, asthma, eczema and so on. I also find that hypnosis can be used to alter the rate of perspiration in someone who is nervous of flying, increase the confidence of those suffering from low self-esteem, and remove the terror some people feel for the hypodermic syringe or dentist's drill.

Doctors and dentists who attend my sessions at the Sandville seem genuinely intrigued by what they observe. Several have commented that the system of induction used by myself is quite different from that practised elsewhere, or even from methods they themselves may have been taught. Traditional induction techniques usually involve some form of visualization, whereas my method concentrates exclusively on memory recall.

Once a satisfactory state of hypnosis has been achieved, patients are in direct communication with the unconscious, much as they are when sleeping. Each is without conscious interference. The essential difference between sleep and self-hypnosis is that during sleep we are not aware of our surroundings and unless some noise disturbs, or danger threatens, the UNS leaves us asleep. In the deep form of self-hypnosis, both minds are aware of the surroundings and the hypnotic state can be self-cancelled whenever the patient so wishes.

While in this deepest state of relaxation, all those who are using it following treatment from myself, will confirm that they cannot be forced to do anything. If they agree with a suggestion, they will act upon it. Otherwise, they will not.

Conscious and unconscious

The elaborate construction of the human brain is a constant source of amazement. I find it remarkable that the part we know as the conscious represents only about one-eleventh of the whole, its sole purpose being to act as a sort of information gatherer, whereas the other ten-elevenths – the UNS – controls much more of our lives than we give it credit for.

How often have you, the motorist, driven for an hour before realizing you cannot remember a thing about the last thirty minutes of your journey? Yet the UNS, like the autopilot it is, clicks into action at the slightest sign of danger, or even suspected danger, such as the wandering of concentration.

What is going on in the minds of people who talk in their sleep? As I see it, this is a case of a dormant conscious having no knowledge of what is being said, because the words are coming direct from the UNS. (Under deep hypnosis' both parts of the mind work simultaneously, so those in that state *do* remember everything when aroused.)

In the state of self-hypnosis, unlike that of sleep-talking (or writing) as already mentioned, the conscious is fully aware of the words emanating from the mind and can be made to understand the meaning behind them. Take Alex B., for example, a family man who worships his wife and three children and would never do anything to harm them. Alex could not comprehend his inner rages when those he loved so much acted against his wishes.

He was never violent towards his family; instead, he focused his outbursts of anger on himself, on one occasion pushing his fist through a plasterboard wall.

His UNS was asked: 'What is the duty of a wife and children?'

'To obey,' came the autocratic response. (This was the voice of his unconscious!)

Who, I wondered, had fed in such a program? The natural assumption that it was his father proved false. Regressed to the time when his mind had been thus programmed, Alex was in the company of Phillip, a brother much older than himself. Phillip had always been a dominant influence in Alex's life; furthermore, he was the type of man who had no time for women or children.

Having established the source of the problem, Alex could see its flaws. Returned to his present age, though still under hypnosis, he was able to view the situation in a different light.

For the benefit of Alex S. and Mandy, his wife, a comparative study was made of the present-day life style of both brothers. Whereas, in adulthood, Alex is enveloped in the love of his family, Phillip can only boast of two failed marriages and a string of failed relationships; his attitude has ruined his own chance of happiness, but why on earth should it continue to threaten that of his brother? Thankfully, it no longer does. The act of comparing the brothers' circumstances changed the program in Alex's mind, with the result that the inner rages no longer occur.

That is why so much of my work is devoted to freeing people from what I call their 'self-imposed chains'. These are just a few of the ways in which self-hypnosis can be seen to activate the healing process.

Notes

1 Troup, John, 'Power of mind over matter', *Wirral News*, 12 June 1986, p.15.
2 Newson, Felicity, 'Living in the past', *Liverpool Echo*, 8 July 1996, p.15.

PART TWO

Their Abilities – Our Memories

3 Biological Tools

Cancer

Cancer: the very word strikes fear and dread in the heart of those affected. To be diagnosed as suffering from any form of the disease represents major trauma. Whatever medical terminology doctors use to wrap it up – malignancy, carcinoma, sarcoma, cancer is still a very frightening condition. In the minds of those affected, fear dominates, because they believe themselves doomed.

While no one would dispute the fact that cancer is a serious, life-threatening disease, it is *not* an automatic death sentence. Like many other right-thinking therapists, I spend considerable time and effort persuading patients of this fact. To be frightened is perfectly understandable, to give up is not. As a matter of interest, more people die of heart attacks and in road traffic accidents than ever do of cancer.

No, I am not claiming to be able to cure this most enigmatic of diseases. All I can offer is to help teach patients to treat themselves in an attempt to reverse its course. Inevitably, some succeed, others do not, and for those who do not it is no reflection on the patients or their families. There are occasions when the path of the disease is so virulent that it has gone beyond being capable of reversal. On the other hand, with those patients who can be helped, I am prepared to devote whatever of my abilities are necessary.

Immune system at work

As already indicated, I believe that when cancer develops it is because our immune system is at fault; in other words, the biological tools that I mentioned earlier are around somewhere, but need to be located and stimulated into action. Those people who enter into a sufficiently deep state of hypnosis can be taught to correct errors in their system; those who do not, can not. Unfortunately, I have no way of predicting which are which, without actually seeing potential patients and testing their response to the hypnotic induction. When basic mechanisms turn normal cells into cancerous ones, they *can* be reversed. Once brain messages are recoded, patients can set about curing themselves.

The comparison with computers has already been made, but for readers unfamiliar with modern technology, here is a different idea. Take the hypothetical case of a managing director who suddenly decided to give his company's maintenance work to the auditors and auditing to the maintenance crew. The result, as we all know, would be chaos. Compare the director to the unconscious mind, his employees to the conscious, and the situation becomes clear. Conscious attempts to take over from the unconscious also result in chaos.

Oddly enough, the problem does not arise in the animal kingdom, because the unconscious part of an animal's mind is allowed to develop naturally and without conscious intervention. It is yet another instance of a so-called *less* intelligent species having *more* intelligent reactions.

Radiation

While I believe that stress is, in some way, connected with cancer, I also believe the disease can be caused, or at least aggravated, by radiation from X-ray machines. When the hydrogen bomb exploded in Hiroshima it killed more than 200,000 people, yet those powerful rays had little or no effect on thousands of survivors. Could the reason be that people's metabolisms have different tolerance levels to radiation? Some of us can have repeated X-rays without ill effects. For others, one dose is enough to spark off a host of problems.

In the days of our grandparents, the only wavelengths passing through the human body were the natural variety (mainly from the sun). In those days, Public Enemy Number One was tuberculosis, not cancer and to anyone interested in TB, I can recommend some excellent reading material.[1] Today, we have an accumulation of man-made emissions to cope with: from gadgets such as radio and television sets, microwave ovens, mobile phones and others too numerous to mention. Is it pure chance that the incidence of cancer has increased so dramatically in recent years? A decade ago, one in ten people worldwide contracted the disease. The figure is now one in three, with one in four deaths attributed to it.

Cancer occurs when cells multiply and grow wildly out of control, when they start destroying healthy tissue. They continue to divide, spread and form new colonies; all the while overwhelming and killing any healthy tissue and organs in their path.

In the early stages of the disease these cells are far too tiny to be visible to the naked eye, yet so powerful that they only have to affect a single cell for that cell to become wildly uncontrolled. Good and bad fuse together until, before we know it, the cancer has grown out of all proportion and the body has been taken over by invading substances of a variety of shapes and form. Unpleasant though the facts may be, I am reliably informed by a surgeon who spends much of his time excising tumours, that forensic examination of those which prove to be malignant has produced some bizarre results. He tells me he has known them to contain fragments of teeth, bone and hair; which rather proves my point about incorrect messages being sent from the brain, or incorrect interpretation of them, once received.

Conventional treatment

After a barrage of tests prove malignancy to be present, patients are usually offered a choice of conventional treatments, none of them pleasant. The offending tumour can either be burned, cut, or poisoned. Hospital staff will not put it so bluntly, of course. They will explain about the need for surgery to remove or reduce the size of the tumour, radiotherapy to slow down its growth, chemotherapy to stop it spreading.

Chemotherapy is sometimes referred to as a drugs cocktail, which sounds palatable, sometimes as cytotoxic drugs, which does not. *Cyto* relates to cells, *toxic* means poison; so, as already indicated, the idea of cytotoxic drugs is to poison malignant cells.

The trouble is that these potent drugs are incapable of discriminating between the normal and the abnormal, with the result that they also poison many perfectly normal, healthy cells. Cancer is easier to prevent than to treat once it has struck. There are distinct advantages in relaxing patients so that their brain messages can be recoded, and their body can set about curing itself.

Retained memories

We know that we have advanced from the first amoebic cell that began life, through every stage of evolution to what we are today. We know, too, that we are capable of retaining the memory of everything contained in the cell given to us by our parents and ultimately using it to our own advantage. Without meaning to be offensive in any way, I venture to suggest that it also shows the production of children to be not so far removed in theory from the production of motor cars.

In the car factory, plans are fed in, parts are placed on a production line, developed, processed and perfected until the finished article emerges: a spanking new vehicle, ready for the road. In human terms, the plans have been fed into the first parental cell, the information they contain enables all the other cells to develop in the body of the growing foetus, until it too emerges as the finished article: a newborn baby, ready for the world.

We take a cutting from something in the garden and grow it on. The resulting plant is identical to that of the parent, but if we cross-fertilize between these two plants, a hybrid results.

Ants, bees and wasps, for example, have used what we now know as cloning techniques since the dawn of time. Given that every cell of our body contains the full program for building any other cell, all it needs is the blueprint. If there were no control over growth, there would be no stable species on earth. Every birth would be a random mutation. But there *is* control, as we can demonstrate in the way the unconscious continues to send its messages around the body.

Across the species, the strong survive because the messages are correct. Gardeners in our midst need no reminding about the dominance of weeds. Allowed to develop, multiply and run rampant, they will soon kill all the surrounding flowers and shrubs. Like the tumour, the weed can be totally unstoppable, choking everything in the vicinity before taking over the entire garden.

To prevent this happening, the first unwanted growth must be pulled up. If that does not work, or if more weeds have already appeared and are shooting up all over the lawn, they can be treated with highly poisonous chemicals.

Methods more friendly to the environment are gradually being introduced by conservationists keen to save the planet. For the sake of humanity, I wish them success. My work with the mind could be compared with eco-friendly methods with the soil. Why cut, burn and bombard with toxic substances if a safer method is available?

Jamie

When cancer has advanced so far that reversal of its progress is no longer possible, the patient can still receive some form of help, as was the case with Jamie, a teenaged patient who made the long and very tiring journey from Scotland to see me. He travelled in the company of his parents and when he arrived at my home it was obvious that he was not long for this world. Jamie was handsome, cheerful and even in his severely weakened state his tall, lithe body showed vestiges of the athlete he once was. Slowly, and with great difficulty, he eased his wasted form into a chair, and began to relax.

The trouble with Jamie was that, despite all the treatment he had already undergone, cancer cells remained in his body and it was distressing for him when the drugs he had been prescribed were so toxic that they were destroying surrounding healthy tissue.

He responded readily to my voice and, in his state of deep hypnosis, this young patient was able to free himself of pain and discomfort and, after proving himself capable of self-treatment, we shook hands, parted company and he promised to let me know how he got on.

I never saw Jamie again. The Christmas card from his father, Bob, explained why. Its message read:

'Sadly, Jamie died on Thursday afternoon, courageous and optimistic to the end. Your help was a great source of strength to him and was still being put into practice right to within 48 hours of his passing. For this, we shall forever be grateful. God Bless.'

There is no way of knowing whether Jamie would have survived had he been treated sooner. Possibly not. His cancer was of such a fast-growing, insidious type that nothing could have prevented the force of its destruction. Yet that boy's life was not wasted. His bravery and stoicism set him apart. I shall continue to remember him fondly.

Sandra P.

It should be clarified here that my case files also contain many unsolicited letters from patients who have been successfully treated. Typical is one received from Sandra P., a young British woman who had taken up residence in Paris, and had heard about my work through regression meetings I once ran in that city.

Sandra explained that she was about to enter hospital for the removal of a large, malignant tumour on her brain and she wondered if hypnosis could do anything to ease the terror she felt at the prospect of what she had been told would be prolonged and painful surgery.

In view of the urgency of the situation I arranged to see her within the week. Sandra, predictably, entered hypnosis without difficulty and began practising self-treatment straight away. I suggested that she should let her doctor know that she planned to use the relaxation techniques I had taught her; not actually for anaesthesia, but for pain relief, relaxation and so on.

The next time I heard from her was in a call from Provence, where she was recuperating. Her voice was full of excitement at the other end of the telephone.

'Remember how terrified I was at the very idea of that operation?' she began. 'Well, I put myself into hypnosis the minute the nurse left me in the ward, and I did it again on the way to theatre.

'After the operation, I was delighted to find I could still do it and I've hardly had any pain at all,' she enthused. 'So thank you very much for helping me. Though it's only ten days since the operation, I already feel healthier than I have for years.'

Sandra added that her doctor was fully in favour. He believed the hypnotic treatment had contributed significantly to her post-operative success and agreed that she should continue with self-treatment as taught.

Self-help groups

Many of my patients have attended or are attending the Sandville. The reason why I see groups of patients there every month is because I believe self-help centres do sterling work helping people suffering from a wide range of health problems. Like many others, these patients have experienced the whole gamut of emotions affecting those who have been diagnosed as suffering from life-threatening illnesses.

Not all of the Sandville's patients have, or have had cancer. Some are suffering from debilitating diseases and conditions such as arthritis, multiple sclerosis, Parkinson's disease, others are recovering from heart attacks and strokes. A third group may be there because of problems related to loneliness, depression, drug addiction, or alcoholism.

Then there are those who may simply be in need of a break from the pressures of caring for a sick or dying relative. The recently bereaved also find their way to this converted farmhouse near the sea.

Practical help for all of these patients comes from teams of volunteers who make themselves available during the day and evening. Volunteers are mostly former cancer sufferers who, after five years without recurrence, have been declared medically free of the disease. Night carers, too, consist of ex-patients, members of their families and retired nurses.

Some of the patients I see at the Sandville are still in the throes of treatment, others are recovering from major illness. In either event, they are only too familiar with the symptoms of nausea, vomiting, fatigue, diarrhoea, infections, bleeding, skin discoloration, as well as hair, appetite and weight loss.

Through self-hypnosis they can eliminate all of these and bring about a general improvement in their condition. By using cards like those referred to in the previous chapter (but specifically designed to treat patients suffering from cancer), they can ensure that, from now on, only malignant cells are affected by the medication.

When the mind is instructed to pass straight through the body any parts of the drug cocktail causing side effects, the body does precisely that. Feelings of nausea and sickness subside, infection and bleeding cease to be a problem, the skin begins to take on a more healthy hue, there is no further hair loss. The appetite increases and patients begin to put on weight. Whether the body actually does pass all the drugs straight through the system or not is something we shall never know.

Cynics might claim that hypnosis merely coincides with spontaneous remission. If that is what they choose to believe, so be it. Belief forms no part of my treatment; my main concern is in seeing an improvement in the patients' health. Cynics can think what they wish. Sometimes doctors refer patients who are deemed terminally ill and no longer respond to conventional forms of treatment. With these patients, as with all the others, the emphasis is on reprogramming their minds, in order, if possible, to cure themselves, but when the condition is too far advanced (as it was with Jamie) then I can at least concentrate on alleviating pain and distress, to help them die with dignity.

An important part of rehabilitating patients by means of self-help is to encourage them to focus on people and events aside from their disease, but no one is ever pressed. Those who wish to retreat into a private corner to be alone with their thoughts are perfectly at liberty to do so. One reason why I feel working at the Sandville to be so worthwhile is because those who visit the centre for treatment manage to call a temporary halt to their own personal problems as they enjoy the company of others: conversing, reading, watching television or strolling around the house and grounds. All do their utmost not to let cancer intrude in their lives, and whether laughter is tense and nervous or the deep and true variety, it matters not. Those who cry a lot also need to laugh a lot and the therapy I give them involves both.

It is not only patients whose pain and distress can be alleviated by self-hypnosis; the technique can also help relieve the stress of nurses and carers whose role it is to deal with those approaching the end of their lives.

Note
1 Ryan, Dr Frank, *Tuberculosis: The Greatest Story Never Told* (Swift Publishers 1992).

4   Losing the Tools

Six cancer patients

William Pearson, Hywel Hopkins, Maureen Arbery, Ethne Parker, Joyce Flower and Tom Evans were all diagnosed as suffering from cancer. Those three men and three women had nothing in common except their illness and the fact that each was referred to the Sandville where, one by one, they gravitated towards my therapy sessions. All had been diagnosed, treated in the conventional manner and were now searching for something else.

William worked on computer systems, Hywel was a professional singer and comedian, Maureen helped her husband Trevor to run their bed and breakfast business, Ethne was a housewife, Joyce was divorced, while Tom was a retired coal miner.

Let them tell their own stories.

William first: 'My world fell apart in February 1988,' he writes 'when I was diagnosed as having testicular cancer. On the eve of my thirty-sixth birthday one of my testicles was surgically removed. In all my life, I never felt so isolated.

'During the days following that operation, no one even mentioned the word (cancer) and I felt as if I had been condemned as unclean. I was totally convinced I was going to die.' He goes on to explain that the one positive thought in his mind was that it was not going to happen in hospital. 'On my return home, Gwyneth Poacher – in her role as Macmillan nurse – came to visit. She explained about her work with cancer patients. That was the first time anyone had mentioned the word, and I was very edgy.'

However, after consultations with an oncologist (cancer specialist) and a Macmillan nurse (also specializing in cancer care) William began to feel some control over his life again. On completion of various tests, doctors assured him that the cancer had not spread and that his chances of survival were very good.

William had been invited to look in on the regular meetings of cancer sufferers and their families, but the idea did not at first appeal.

'I didn't want to mix with people who were dying. That, I am now very ashamed to say, was how I felt.'

In the spring of 1992 he changed his mind, deciding to pay a one-off visit to the centre without committing himself to anything. However, in the informal environment he immediately relaxed and decided he did want to visit on a regular basis after all. Meeting and befriending other patients and their families, William could see the need for volunteer work not just with his new friends but on the property, in the garden and elsewhere. He added his name to the list of volunteers prepared to make tea, serve in the bar, ferry patients to and from hospital or to connect with public transport. As the centre's project manager, he made himself responsible for erecting all the shelves and ensuring that the refurbishments, generally, were in order.

'To realize that other people have had similar problems and are still enjoying life is a great inspiration,' he reflects. 'The Sandville, I soon realized, was not a place where people came to die: but to live.

'Unfortunately, not all those you get to know survive and it is particularly hard not to become too emotionally close to other residents. Losing friends is an incredibly painful experience and can make coping very difficult.'

William's words are extracted from the centre's newsletter, of which he is editor. It was during a particularly difficult period in the summer of 1992 that he first came to my attention and we shall follow his progress shortly, but first, let us move on to the next patient.

Hywel Hopkins' trouble was not unlike that of William. Hywel was earning his living as a comedian, but was not amused when, in June 1985, his right testicle became inflamed and swollen. 'I thought it was a double hernia,' he recalls. The doctor he consulted thought otherwise and within a week admitted Hywel to hospital, where he was horrified at the diagnosis of testicular cancer.

Apparently the condition occurs mainly in young men though, thankfully, it is fairly rare. Nevertheless, doctors do advise young men to make regular examination of the testicles, a practice they consider as important as breast self-examination in women. It makes sense not to ignore lumps, swellings and other enlargements, because the sooner trouble is detected, the better the chance of successful treatment. William and Hywel sensibly had their condition investigated at the earliest possible stage.

Hywel's testicle was surgically removed and the operation was followed by six months of chemotherapy. But there was more trouble in store. The patient himself takes up the story:

'A year after the first batch of trouble showed up, I had another shock when my left eye went scarlet, then a huge area underneath went black.'

Because of the pain and inflammation, Hywel was admitted to hospital once more, this time for a brain scan. Yet, despite his intensive questioning, he says nobody would confirm his suspicions that this too was cancer.

'They opened me up, but found it impossible to reach the source of the trouble, telling me later that if they made one false move my brain could be affected.

'The tests were completed, I was invited back to hospital and informed that another operation was necessary. It saved my life, but left me blind in one eye for ten weeks. That little episode was followed by four weeks of radiotherapy and six months' chemotherapy.'

Hywel had certainly had his share of problems. Recovering from the shock of what he had been through would take time and it was to be another five years before his case was brought to my attention. By then (June, 1991), he had been given a clean bill of health, but was still very traumatized.

★

Maureen Arbery's breast lump had been present for a year before it was diagnosed as cancerous. Because it had not been deemed malignant, Maureen carried on with her busy life; coping with her family, the business, and with Trevor's intermittent bouts of depression.

In January 1991 she entered hospital for surgery to have the lump and its surrounding glands removed. The operation was followed by a course of radiotherapy and five years later she too was declared free of disease, as patients routinely are if they remain symptom-free for that length of time.

Latest statistics[1] show that one in twelve women in the UK develops breast cancer at some time in her life, and it is much more common in women over the age of fifty.

By means of breast screening (at designated hospitals and health centres) it is possible to find small changes in the breast before any other signs of cancer manifest themselves. Again, if these are found early enough, there is a good chance for the patient.

On being diagnosed as suffering from ovarian cancer, Ethne Parker describes the effect on her system as *devastating*. In common with many others suffering from such a condition, her first reaction was that she was going to die.

'Then I agreed to take part in trials of a new drug,' she recalls. 'On completion of the trials, I wasn't sure where to turn.'

In the event, Ethne turned to the Sandville, where it was suggested that she should try some of the complementary treatments on offer. She surveyed the list of those available and decided to start off with reflexology.

This is a means of 'diagnosing' and treating patients by exploring the feet and massaging the relevant areas. Reflexologists work on the assumption that a series of energy channels run to the feet from all over the body.

As a result, when troubled areas are found in parts of the feet, the relevant parts of the body are deemed to be malfunctioning.

Once any blockages in the energy channels have been detected, reflex areas of the foot are massaged and compressed in order to clear those blockages. The therapist then attempts to stimulate the body's own healing forces into action.

Because the aim of the reflexologist is to tone and harmonize the energy flow throughout the patient's body, his technique can complement my own. It is actually a very pleasant procedure and Ethne tells me she found it both calming and relaxing. But she still felt the need to try something else.

Hypnotherapy had also been suggested to her, but, having no experience of it, she was not sure whether she wanted to try the technique or not. Frankly, at that stage, she did not think it would do her any good.

After a routine cervical smear, Joyce Flower's initial reaction was to ignore the request to return for a further consultation. It is not unusual (though, in my opinion, perfectly understandable) for a woman to panic on receiving such a letter from a hospital clinic.

Only in Joyce's case the reaction was not one of panic but of disbelief; as she recalls:

'When they said I had cancer, I was convinced they'd got it wrong. But they gave it to me straight. With treatment, I had a ninety per cent chance of survival. Without treatment? They couldn't say.'

Her own doctor told her not to worry unduly, since the lump had been found at such an early stage, but by then she was terrified. Having had time to reflect, she did not like the thoughts preoccupying her mind. She describes them graphically:

'Four of my friends had died of cancer in the last few years. Now it looked like my number was up too: electric chair . . . curtains . . . the end of the line.

'And yet, something inside me said I wasn't ready for a wing-fitting. I'd gone through rough patches before and come out smiling. I'd manage again, somehow. I'm a survivor.'

She certainly is. Married too young, Joyce remained married only for the sake of the children, but eventually, at the age of forty-seven, having successfully raised her family, she was divorced and ready to 'find herself'. She returned to full-time education, passed several examinations, took driving lessons and developed a host of new hobbies.

'Having regained some of my old confidence and self-esteem, I went back-packing in Australia and Thailand, then set out on several other adventures.'

The cancer diagnosis was a bombshell and the resultant depression hit her hard.

'When I was really down in the dumps one day, someone a lot wiser than myself pointed out that it's not the occurrence of an illness that matters, but how you deal with it. That's been my motto ever since.

'At first, when I was admitted to hospital, I was scared stiff and wanted to hide away. I wouldn't mix with anyone.

'Then, one day, another patient got me to stop referring to my condition in hushed tones, describing it as a *problem* or even *Big C*. She made me face up to the fact that I had cancer. It didn't have to be a killer, she kept saying, and she repeated the words so often I began to convince myself she was right.'

Joyce arrived at the Sandville not knowing what to expect.

'I wondered where all the people suffering from cancer were,' she muses. 'It was only later I discovered them all around me, but I didn't realize it. Through self-help, they were coming to terms with their condition and fighting it.

'That made me realize I wasn't so vulnerable, or pathetic after all. The people I met were not all cancer patients, anyway. They were suffering from all sorts of chronic and debilitating diseases. They were people in crisis, because that's what the Sandville is: a crisis centre.

'Through sharing mutual problems, caring, releasing emotions, deep friendships are struck up. Patients do unburden themselves, but they laugh and joke a lot too.

'The camaraderie, the joy, the general buzz of the place got to me straight away. It was plain to see that it inspired everyone who came.'

Joyce goes on to explain that (like William) before she knew what was happening involvement with others had enabled her to stop feeling sorry for herself. It is not unusual for those who have recovered from potentially life-threatening illnesses to become volunteer workers at the centre where they themselves have been helped. Joyce was only too eager to join their ranks.

By the time I met her she was happily settled in: like one of the family, almost. The only problem now was that the strain of caring for so many sick people was causing her considerable stress. Unlike Ethne, Joyce had no doubt at all that hypnotherapy would help her. She was one of the first to step forward.

Tom Evans had been a miner since the age of fourteen, eventually acquiring his own small mine in the valleys. Long hours of work underground and little time for relaxation gradually took their toll. His health began to suffer, until, in 1970, spinal arthritis forced him to close the mine.

Two years later his wife Val resumed her nursing career. Val continued in her profession until 1990, when his condition began to deteriorate rapidly. This time, the diagnosis was cancer. Val explains the details: 'A mass on the oesophagus had travelled to the stomach and a lengthy operation was necessary to remove it. Surgery also involved the removal of ribs, deflation of a lung, and the widening of his gullet.'

Tom recovered from the operation but, with his stomach reduced considerably in size, it became necessary for Val to feed him five times daily, with the type of bland and boring meals he hated.

'It was a time of loneliness and uncertainty, but Tom was still with me and that was all that mattered.'

With hindsight, Val confesses that her biggest mistake in those days was her reluctance to make her husband aware of the nature of his condition.

'Knowing the type of man he was, I believed he would have given up rather than become a burden so I gave him what I considered to be the best care humanly possible. I thought I was mothering him, but I was actually smothering him. I was taking away his dignity and his will to fight.'

Too proud to accept help, Val was making herself ill in the process. She freely admits that it was not until the Macmillan nurse assigned to Tom drew the situation to her attention that she began to see sense. A visit to the Sandville was suggested.

'Tom's nurse told me of the various therapies on offer and promised that the whole atmosphere of the place would be a great help to him. She thought a break there wouldn't do me any harm either.'

In June 1993, the Sandville's new extension, housing the purpose-built therapy suite, was officially opened by Her Royal Highness the Duchess of Kent. Sister Poacher had met the duchess during a television programme in which they were both guests. The duchess, having expressed interest in the various aspects of self-help, was invited to pay a visit and meet some of those involved. When she accepted the invitation, everyone at the centre was delighted.

On the day in question, the royal visitor was most enthusiastic about the project and all those connected with it. She met the teams of professional carers, spoke to therapists, volunteers and those of the patients who were well enough to be presented to her. Val recalls what happened during the informal moments after the ceremony: 'When the duchess was told that Tom had cancer, she introduced him to Joe and left them together.'

It was clear that Tom was very ill, but I was immediately impressed by his personality and his sheer enthusiasm for living. The severity of his condition had done nothing to dampen his spirits; nor, indeed, his sense of fun. He was a small man, slightly built, but with a huge personality. He had a spontaneous sense of humour and kept us enthralled with his lively repertoire of jokes and stories.

On top of all that, he was blessed – like so many of his compatriots – with a splendid singing voice. On my subsequent visits, when Tom was in residence, there were no prizes for guessing the source of those lovely songs from the valleys. They were pure joy to listen to.

I find it quite remarkable how he managed to surround himself with so much joy and sunshine. Strangers, or anyone unaware of his condition, would never suspect he was terminally ill.

So there we had it: six patients whom Fate had decreed should converge at the Sandville. All wanted to be taught self-hypnosis, in order to reprogram their minds for the benefit of their bodies. How would they cope?

Would William accept the ever-present problem surrounding him? Or would he prove overburdened by the effects of losing more new-found friends from the disease which could so easily have claimed himself?

Would Hywel escape further unpleasant experiences of pain and trauma and be able to resume his career?

Would Maureen continue to be symptom-free and live to see her young children grow up?

Would Ethne stop being afraid of hypnosis and give it a chance?

Would Joyce be able to continue looking after others in the way she wanted, or would the strain eventually take its toll?

And Tom . . . when the stories had all been told and the ballads been sung, would he prove too ill even to enter hypnosis; or, if he were to succeed in entering deeply enough for treatment, would he be able to remove − or at least slow down − the course of his disease by having the strengths of his unconscious added to his fight?

In the next chapter answers to these and other questions will be provided as we follow the progress of all six.

First, though, let me explain something of the circumstances under which I work. What I like to do is sit patients in a comfortable chair with head support, rather than have them lie on a couch. I do not lower the lights or draw the curtains, but sit alongside or opposite them in order to watch out for the flickering eye movement which precedes entry into the first stage of hypnosis. I speak in a quietly persuasive monotone (patients have described my voice as 'pleasant, soothing, confident') until my trained eye can see that they are beginning to respond. Various inflexions are used for the induction and deepening of hypnosis; the actual words and their implications are also relevant. By softly intoning instructions to rest, to drift into a state of relaxation and so on, I can soon tell what depth each patient has reached.

There are various stages or levels of hypnosis. The first involves a noticeable upward turning of the eyes when the lids begin to flutter, then involuntarily close.

Rapid eye movement (REM) follows; this indicates true hypnosis and continues until the person being treated is guided down into deeper levels of relaxation. In normal sleep, the first REM period does not appear until after about thirty minutes of slow wave (non-REM) sleep. The rapid eye movement in ordinary sleep is assumed to be accompanied by vivid dreaming and loss of muscle tone; for the person under hypnosis the effect is quite the opposite in that it marks the beginning of the flooding back of auditory, visual and tactile memories (which will be explained in later chapters). During the second and third stages of hypnosis patients enter deeper and deeper levels until, down at the fourth stage, it becomes possible to practise hypnotic analgesia and anaesthesia.

By the time the patient has reached this level I know that the conscious part of the mind has been shut down and I have established a direct link through to the unconscious — that part which motivates people's vital processes even though they are not necessarily aware of its existence. This is the point at which I arouse those primitive defence mechanisms in the body which were once a built-in part of the human metabolism but which, over thousands of years, have atrophied and ceased to function.

The idea that people under hypnosis are asleep in the usual sense of the word and are unaware of their surroundings could stem from the fact that, in Hollywood film representations of hypnosis, the operator was invariably seen to induce amnesia so that those under hypnosis were unaware of what was happening when they were allegedly 'out cold'.

The patient, in the story-line, could then get away with the proverbial murder. After all, he did not know what he was doing, did he? Nonsense. No one can be made to do anything under hypnosis that they would not do in their waking state, but if, in their waking state, they wanted to commit a specific crime then the answer would be different.

Why, then, must the eyes be shut? The reason is simply because, if they remain open, attention can wander and it is important for patients' health that their minds are focused exclusively on what my voice is saying to them. There must be no confusion filtering through to the unconscious mind.

Note
1 'NHS Breast Screening, The Facts', Health Education Authority leaflet (1997).

PART THREE

When Hypnotherapy can Help

5   Rediscovering the Tools

William Pearson

In the days before William had been given his clean bill of health
Sister Poacher and her team at the Sandville had helped him face
his fears. They had supported him through some trying times and
given him that all-important positive attitude. His malignant
tumour and the effects of the treatment had already been attended
to but now, in the aftermath, reaction was beginning to set in.
William's initial request for hypnotherapy came in the summer of
1992, when he was feeling low and needed a good morale-boost.
At the back of his mind was the ever-present fear that his cancer
might return.

Anxiety is not uncommon in such circumstances. Patients who
have had what they consider to have been a brush with death do
sometimes feel depressed, and who can blame them? William
needed to be convinced that his problems were in the past.
Consciously, he was coping; but his unconscious mind needed that
extra push: hence the request for hypnosis. To his credit, he
responded readily and reached the deepest level without difficulty;
enabling me to reinforce all that had been said before.

I also instructed his immune system to prevent any recurrence
of his cancer and, in line with what others had told him, stressed
the importance of a positive attitude. With control of his UNS, he
had the ability to cope with further bouts of anxiety and depression, thus giving himself a better chance of remaining fit and well.

Hywel Hopkins, Maureen Arbery

Hywel and Maureen also responded readily to the hypnotic induction, both proving to be fast learners and promising to practise the self-hypnotic technique as taught. Each had been declared free of cancer and for the benefit of those who might wonder why they continued to frequent the self-help centre Hywel provides the answer. When anger and fear take over, he says, it is helpful to meet other patients at various stages of their disease and its treatment. For Hywel the comparison of experiences and progress is mutually beneficial.

Maureen puts it another way:

'In spite of all the suffering and distress people here might be going through, it's an incredibly happy environment. You'd be amazed at how attitudes to life change when you've had cancer. Ours certainly has.'

Ethne Parker

Ethne still had doubts but, at the suggestion of friends, decided to look in on a therapy session.

She freely admits that, when she first observed people undergoing hypnosis, she was sceptical. She believed that, in order to please me, they were putting on an act: in a sense *performing* as they might on stage.

Let her take up the story: 'I watched a lady being helped into her chair and could hardly believe the evidence of my own eyes when, after that one treatment, she got up and marched away. It was an immediate improvement; quite amazing, Then my turn came round.'

There was no one more surprised than Ethne herself at her swift response, although when I believed her sufficiently relaxed to begin the healing process it was *my* turn to be surprised. Ethne recounts what happened:

'In my state of light hypnosis, I could hear Joe talking to my husband, Ralph, about possible side effects of the treatment I was having at the hospital, one of them being hair loss. Overhearing those two words I felt myself freeze. It was as if the very idea had turned on a tap inside my head and the tears began to flow.'

Ethne's reaction was spontaneous and unpredictable, yet not altogether surprising in the circumstances, though I was unaware of it at the time. I asked her – while still under hypnosis – if the thought of hair loss worried her. She made no reply but became so agitated that I felt the need to relax her and bring her out of hypnosis.

Only then did I learn why this patient had reacted so strongly to those two words. Ethne was a former wig-maker and this made the cause of her distress abundantly clear.

It will be recalled (chapter 2) that during the hypnotic induction I make a point of telling the patient that if I inadvertently say anything which upsets or disturbs them, they will cancel the hypnotic state. The very mention of the words 'hair loss' was almost enough to bring Ethne out of hypnosis. Treated successfully for her fear, she was taught self-hypnosis and I am pleased to say everything worked out satisfactorily.

What I did not realize when I first met Ethne was that she had already lost her hair and was wearing a wig, albeit one which had been designed so skilfully that none but the most perceptive observer would be aware of it. Nevertheless, her lack of hair represented Ethne's 'achilles heel'. It is hardly surprising, therefore, that she was feeling so sensitive and vulnerable.

Loss of hair (medically known as alopaecia), is demoralizing, particularly for a woman. Regrowth of hair will occur spontaneously after chemotherapy, and sometimes after alopaecia from other causes, yet patients can also be successfully treated for the condition by hypnosis. Regrowth after hypnosis starts fairly soon and the first batches of hair to push through are not unlike the soft down on a baby's head. Sometimes, the new crop is curlier than before, at other times more straight; there may also be colour variations. But patients are usually so pleased with its very presence that they seldom worry about form, texture, or colour.

It might be appropriate to mention here that, on a subsequent visit to the Sandville, I hardly recognized Ethne. She looked somehow very different. I could not quite place what it was: she seemed prettier, more attractive and generally much younger. Not being the type of individual who makes personal comments, I declined to voice my thoughts straight away.

Ethne caught the quizzical expression on my face whenever I glanced in her direction: 'You keep looking at me,' she stated and before I had a chance to apologize for what might have been interpreted as rudeness, her face lit up. 'Yes, it's me, Ethne. And it's all my own. My hair . . . it's regrown since you taught me self-hypnosis. I don't need my wig any more.'

Joyce Flower

Joyce, like Ethne, had little knowledge of hypnosis, also associating it with stage and screen shows. Until we met she knew nothing of its potential for healing.

'I never realized people could be given the opportunity to control their own minds,' she reflects. 'It's remarkable the way virtually anyone can be taught to treat themselves.'

Joyce graphically describes how she felt during the induction: 'I became aware of every muscle relaxing, every anxiety floating away. Even the old wrinkles seemed to be ironing themselves out. The hypnotic state was quite fantastic: like being in an air bubble. It was a state of inner peace.'

Joyce needed no encouragement to practise every day; she had already made up her mind to do so!

'I don't want to lose the ability. I should imagine it's like playing a musical instrument. Keep at it, or you'll soon get rusty.'

The question thus arises why, if patients have been given the ability to treat themselves do they need to keep seeing me? In theory, they do not, or should not. In practice, follow-up visits to Sandville patients enables me to monitor their progress.

It is natural for those who have suffered from cancer to worry about the possibility of recurrence; though doctors do generally believe that if patients have been free of disease for five years they are likely to remain free indefinitely. Before the five-year period has expired, former sufferers usually submit themselves to screening tests, so that any further hint of trouble can be dealt with immediately.

These high-tech methods of screening for cancerous and precancerous changes in the body are all very well, but surely nature can do it better? I believe that, spurred into action, the body's own immune system has the potential to do exactly the same; more, quite probably, by recognizing malignant cells which might confuse even the most sophisticated man-made machine. I am given to understand that some of those rogue cells are so similar to healthy ones as to be virtually indistinguishable from them.

The immune system, with the correct program fed into its own detection agency, is well equipped to pinpoint anything about to go wrong in our vital organs and tissues, however small, however well masked it might be. That is why, even when patients have recovered from their respective illnesses and are to all intents and purposes fit and well, the instructions to the UNS continue to be reinforced.

Tom Evans

Val confesses to having felt very apprehensive at the prospect of her sick husband being hypnotized. Never having encountered the phenomenon in her nursing career, she too was under the impression that its purpose was to make fools of people; or, at least, encourage them to make fools of themselves.

'I had no idea the technique could be used therapeutically,' she remarked and was therefore astonished to observe Tom's swift response.

After seeing how much he had benefited from the treatment, she was eager to try it for herself, which she did, successfully. Val had been in the habit of taking pills for tension headaches, but after one session she stopped, determined to use self-hypnosis instead.

During the course of the next few months, I gave her husband several treatments and we became firm friends. As Tom's illness progressed, he needed several sessions of hypnosis to help him cope, not just with the cancer itself but with associated stress and anxiety. Depression and malaise are understandable in cancer sufferers. So, too, are feelings of loneliness and loss.

The side-effects of radiotherapy may also need counteracting. Patients undergoing this form of treatment are likely to suffer tiredness and nausea. They also usually have something resembling sunburn on the site of the area being radiated, which renders that area very sensitive to the touch. Through self-hypnosis, all these matters can be dealt with.

Pain control is another important aspect of patient care and, as far as hypnotherapy is concerned, it matters not whether the pain is from the primary site of the cancer, or from secondary growths. Provided the patient learns the technique and puts it into practice, control should result.

Sometimes patients need hypnotherapy between my monthly visits, and those who feel up to making the five-hundred-mile round trip between South Wales and Merseyside do so. For the benefit of those too weak to travel and in urgent need of treatment, I have devised a scheme whereby Sister Poacher can do my work by proxy, so to speak.

It works like this: when I have inducted the patient into hypnosis and am satisfied that the UNS is receptive to instructions I tell him, or her, to respond to a pre-determined code-word or series of numbers provided by Sister Poacher (the post-hypnotic signal, briefly referred to in the previous chapter).

Out of hypnosis I test the method and, once I know it is working correctly, ask Sister Poacher to put it into action. When the response is correct, that patient can be helped to manage any crisis which may arise in my absence.

The technique has proved invaluable on many occasions and saves those who are deeply troubled having to wait for my next visit. When I am actually at the centre, booster or 'top-up' treatments are given where necessary.

Tom was one man who benefited greatly from the scheme. As he became increasingly ill, and needed more hypnosis to help him manage his pain and distress, Sister Poacher was able to provide it. Much as I should like to have seen my friend on a regular weekly basis, the geographical distance between us made it impossible.

What happened was that whenever he was feeling in need of

some extra help, if Sister Poacher was on hand she would provide it personally. If she was not immediately available Val would telephone from her husband's bedside and place the receiver in a position where he could listen to her voice in comfort. Within seconds, the coded message would have the effect of easing away Tom's troubles and enabling him to drift off into a deep, pain-free sleep.

No one should have to endure pain when it is possible to switch it off. When I was at the centre, I always gave Tom priority treatment. We would sit and chat for a while: sometimes about his physical, psychological or emotional problems: sometimes about none of those. Even at the most advanced stage of his illness, this remarkable man could still rustle up the energy to reminisce about the good times in his life and his marriage, and to crack the odd joke.

Once he began to relax, he found the prescribed medication more tolerable and in the moments when he was attacked by stress and anxiety, the act of voicing his fears eliminated them. He assured me the newly devised scheme also helped him sleep comfortably on those nights when pain might have overwhelmed him.

The idea, devised for Tom, has worked equally well for others. The concept of calling upon Sister Poacher's aid has helped a variety of patients suffering from conditions other than cancer. This form of treatment can be spread over a period of days, or weeks, to suit individual needs. In anguish, in agony, or despair, it matters not: if sufferers can be helped by this means, they are. All they have to do, is ask.

Extending the service?
Would it not be simpler to extend the service by using tape-recorded messages for general distribution instead, one might ask? After all, other therapists sell such tapes in their thousands.

Accepting that self-hypnosis tapes are widely available, I am not in favour of them. I believe it is essential actually to meet patients first and induct them into hypnosis on a one-to-one basis, because only then is it possible to determine whether the response is correct. The other point on which I feel strongly is the ever-present possibility of emotional dependency. There are very real dangers here.

It is vitally important that patients do not become dependent on my voice, or on anyone else's other than Sister Poacher's, under the given conditions. Nor should they feel the need to depend on someone's tape-recorded words. Independence is what this treatment is all about: controlling your *own* mind for your *own* ends.

You, the patient, hold the key. You are the only one who can unlock the door and, having opened up, are the only one who should be in there, in control. As I see it, there is yet another inherent danger with hypnotic tapes. I have already pointed out that I always instruct the UNS never to allow that person to fall asleep at the wheel of a car or any other vehicle they might happen to be driving. The practice of listening to tapes while cruising along miles of motorway is too commonplace for comfort. Listen to music, radio programmes and talking books by all means, but one needs little imagination to suppose what might happen if one of those do-it-yourself hypnotic tapes were mixed in with the others?

A smile costs nothing

From all of this it can be seen that hypnotherapy is not a form of treatment to be feared, but mental attitude is also important. A happy, cheery person is more likely to be healthy than someone who is depressed; and, if health is no longer good, being happy and cheerful does help to keep problems at bay.

Depression and misery increase stress levels: laughter lessens them – and I am not the only person who holds this view. Let me tell you about a young couple of my acquaintance who were going through a particularly bad patch. I shall call them Gina and Andy, though those are not their names. Gina was thirty-nine, Andy forty-two and Gina had cancer. Despite the many operations she had endured to remove deep-seated tumours, the cancer was still invading her body.

After numerous recurrences of malignancy the quality of Gina's life was so poor and her medication so strong that she needed daily treatment in hospital. There was also the dressing of an open wound to be attended to.

Andy, while trying to hold down a demanding job, was anxious and exhausted. He was doing his best to cope but the strain of it all was weighing him down. In the belief that a short break was all they needed to give them the incentive to go on, Gina and Andy visited the Sandville. The centre had been recommended to them by nursing staff at the hospital. There would, they were assured, be ample opportunity for mixing with others in the same situation. The exercise, fresh air and companionship would do them good. Gina's clinician arranged for a district nurse to administer the daily medication and dress the wound.

With so much help on hand, the couple had no need to feel embarrassed at having to allow others to take over the most basic tasks. They would enjoy it, they were assured. And yes, they were determined to do so. They looked upon it as a holiday; never having had one since their honeymoon.

On arrival, Gina and Andy – each being blessed with a happy-go-lucky type of nature – gave the impression of not having a care in the world. They integrated well and were liked by almost everyone they met. I use the word 'almost' deliberately.

One elderly woman, mistaking the pair for visitors, resented their lively presence and wondered what gave them the right to be so carefree. She found them much too exuberant for her taste.

'Must you laugh so much?' her tone was haughty. 'Don't you realize there are sick people here?' She paused, to give her next statement dramatic effect.

'I have *cancer.*' The way she uttered the word implied it was something to be acknowledged and revered.

'Me, too,' quipped Gina, as nonchalantly as she could manage.

For a moment the older woman was rendered speechless. Then she repeated her question: 'So why do you laugh and joke so much?'

This time, the answer came from Andy, who resented the woman's still-underlying hostility and did not mince his words:

'Because if we didn't, we'd be crying. There are two problems with crying. One is that when you start it's not easy to stop. The other is that if you go around moping you make everyone around you miserable too. And that's not fair. Laughing isn't easy; but it's worth the effort. When you laugh you forget your troubles.'

The older woman's reaction is not on record. She might have been interested to know that once the young couple were in the privacy of their room, or strolling hand in hand along the beach, well away from the other guests, the tears came. And when they did they flowed copiously.

We must not pre-judge. There may have been a valid reason for the older woman's attitude. Her tension may well have been due to the fact that she had only recently been diagnosed, and had not yet adjusted to the shock. Those who work as professional diagnosticians tell me they find that a diagnosis of cancer affects patients differently.

The initial reaction for some is to break down and sob pitifully, while others put on a brave face; a third group develop an ostrich attitude: by burying their head in the sand they pretend the tumour is not there, that it will go away. Whatever the sentiments, it is apparently some considerable time before acceptance sets in. In the intervening period, cancer sufferers often feel resentful towards those they perceive as fit and healthy. The elderly woman had clearly mistaken Gina's radiation burns for sunburn acquired in some exotic holiday resort and resented her apparent well-being. That was a pity, because it created immediate tension between them, something of which patients suffering from cancer need no extra helpings.

To return to our original six: William, Hywel, Maureen, Ethne, Joyce and Tom. All had had their immune systems aroused. They had found, polished up and reactivated their biological tools. The question now was, would they continue to use them, in other words, to practise self-hypnosis, as taught?

That was something only they could decide. The wheels had been set in motion, it was up to each individual to exploit their new-found mental abilities. Placed in the driving seat of their lives, they were in control not only of the vehicles but of the road ahead, however long or short that road might prove.

Their case histories will be concluded in the next chapter.

6 Using Them Again

William

Ten years have now elapsed since William was diagnosed as suffering from testicular cancer, three since doctors gave him the all clear, and six since his first session of hypnotherapy. I am happy to report that, at the time of writing, William is fit and well. In the wake of his illness, he practises self-hypnosis to prevent the return of his cancer, as well as for relaxation and sleep. 'My general health has improved and I feel better than I ever did,' he remarks. 'It's incredible to think what can be achieved after just one treatment.' Today, William's spare time is devoted to the interests of others. Apart from editing and writing almost every page of the Sandville's newsletter, he is currently chairman of the Foundation's executive committee.

Hywel

Hywel is also keeping healthy and has resumed his stage career, albeit with a different emphasis. Concentrating now on charity performances, he raises funds for a variety of good causes, mainly related to the self-help centre. Thankfully, he has had no recurrence of his problem. Doctors specializing in the treatment of testicular cancer tell me that this particular form of the disease is the most common cancer in young men and usually occurs between the ages of fifteen and fifty. If detected early enough, survival rate is excellent.

Patients who have gone five years without a recurrence are given the all clear and that, say former sufferers, is when those moments of absolute terror give way to overwhelming relief. If testicular cancer is left untreated, the picture is grim. For those interested in this particular topic literature is freely available. The Imperial Cancer Research Fund has produced a most informative booklet.[1] With its whimsical title *A Whole New Ball Game*, it is intended to catch the attention of men in the age-group most likely to be affected. It is, nevertheless, full of important facts and figures about testicular cancer.

Maureen

Maureen is well and happy; self-hypnosis has become a routine part of her life.

'I've been doing it successfully since six months after the operation and practise it every day; more often if I'm stressed-out, or lacking in confidence,' she tells me. 'It gives me a great mental lift.'

Maureen was declared free of cancer in January, 1996. She and Trevor still visit the Sandville on a regular basis; she, to see the many friends they have both made there; he, to 'recharge his batteries'. 'It's remarkable how people's attitude to life changes when they've had cancer,' she reflects. 'Ours certainly has.'

Ethne

Ethne has been back to hospital for various health checks since that original diagnosis; again, everything seems fine. As I write, this patient is in remission and things are looking up.

She uses hypnotherapy and reflexology to help improve the quality of her life, finding the latter form of treatment highly effective in easing constipation caused by the prescribed medication. Howard Plummer, the centre's senior tutor in reflexology[2] echoes my own sentiments about enlisting the aid of others when he is unable to attend to them personally. He has, therefore, taught the basics of his technique to Ethne's husband, Ralph.

Ethne is fortunate in that Ralph has recently retired from the police force, so has sufficient time on his hands to be able to help her on a regular basis.

'Joe and Howard are both very sensitive,' reflects Ethne. 'Just as

Joe picked up on my dread of hair-loss, Howard was able to tell me that, while receiving chemotherapy, I was blocked in the area of my colon. It's remarkable how information like that can be detected from touching areas of the feet. A hospital consultant subsequently confirmed Howard's thoughts and I was given a barium enema, which located the problem.' Ethne and Ralph are lavish in their praise of the self-help treatments available and firmly believe in the ability of the mind to heal bodily ills. 'I lead a full and good life,' concludes Ethne. 'If I hadn't been led here, I would probably spend my time curled up on the settee at home, crying my life away.'

Joyce

Joyce, too, is making excellent progress. With her illness firmly lodged on the back burner of her memory, she neither forgets nor dwells on it. Her life is too busy for idle speculation about what might have been.

Always one for learning new skills and giving of herself to others, she decided to train as a professional carer and, having successfully completed the course, she now spends much of her time helping the seriously ill. Why did she want to volunteer her services in this way?

Let Joyce herself answer that question: 'I'd been through serious domestic problems, battled with a life-threatening illness, gone back to school and travelled half-way round the world, so had considerable experience of life.

'It meant that I could relate to more people than I could have done five or ten years earlier.'

Joyce is only too familiar with the severe mental and emotional strain resulting from screening tests to determine the presence or otherwise of cancer. She knows, too, that when malignancy is confirmed, if the strain is not to bring on despondency the sufferer needs to have a sympathetic listener close by. Otherwise, mental breakdown could render the patient virtually incapable of fighting the disease.

Some people find it easier to talk than others. While one type of patient may have an immediate urge to open up and let it all pour out, another may be stunned into silence. A third group may have been brought up not to discuss their problems with others and are seriously repressed because of their upbringing. This does not render the silent sufferers any more capable of shrugging off their problems. The quietest, the most private, individuals can be sorely in need of emotional support. They may not show it, but they can be just as vulnerable as the others. Even today, a belief that cancer is something to be ashamed of is not unusual.

Skilled indeed is the observer who can recognize and cope with the many signs and symptoms. Having someone on hand to guide the way has been found to be a great help. Allowing people to share their emotional burden can make sufferers feel their lives have been handed back. In terms of hypnosis, teaching them to control their unconscious mind ensures that they keep those lives strong and healthy. Another important factor is having someone ready and willing to help in times of crisis.

When I cannot be there myself to ensure that patients are in a sufficiently deep state of hypnosis to bring about the type of relaxation they need, a 'proxy' therapist is the next best thing. As an emergency procedure, it works very well. Joyce is one woman who is utterly convinced of its effectiveness:

'That idea about Gwyneth being able to use Joe's methods to help anyone in trouble when he's not here himself, works very well,' she says. 'Sometimes, when people are in trouble and need to get back to their place of inner peace, they find they're too tense to manage on their own.

'But it's important for them to lower their stress levels, so Gwyneth uses Joe's code-words or numbers to relax them. I've seen several patients respond to her voice in the same way that they do to his and the result is just as if he were here in person.'

Tom

Sadly, Tom's story has a less happy ending than those of the other five in the group. The outlook for this patient never was very optimistic. He was already desperately ill when we first met and I am afraid death was inevitable.

When it happened Val and Gwyneth were there to comfort him in his passing. Shortly afterwards Val reflected on the events of that dark day in January 1996:

'Between them, Joe and Gwyneth gave Tom a new quality of life. And they gave him hope, something not available anywhere else. When it was time for him to go, it was easier than it might have been. He'd been given the strength to live and now he had the strength to die. I firmly believe that he had four extra years of life because of what he gained at the Sandville. The end came peacefully.'

Despite the fact that Tom had been ill for many years, his death was still a very great shock to Val, who grieved deeply. In the early days of her widowhood she could not face returning to her empty home, choosing instead to stay on at the centre for a period of respite care.

When her family joined her she drew comfort from their presence, but her closeness to Tom left her feeling lost. Under hypnosis I fed the message into her unconscious mind that, if she were not to be overwhelmed by gloom, she needed to keep her conscious mind occupied. The practice of hypnosis helped her cope and gave her the incentive to go on. In time, she began to adapt to her changed circumstances and began to look forward rather than back.

Like Joyce and others before her, she trained as a carer and became a regular volunteer at the centre which had become the focus of her life. As a result, she has been able to return some of the love and devotion given to her when she was the one in need.

Knowing the agony of nursing a partner through terminal illness, she found herself in a strong position to offer support to others undergoing a similar experience. She, above all, could empathize with those weighed down by the burden of responsibility and comfort them in their anguish. In helping so many people through their painful experiences, Val has begun to find personal rewards. By allowing those in trouble to unburden themselves of their misery she is fulfilling a real need. Val experienced cancer at close hand, and therefore believes she has a special bond with others in the same situation.

'Helping others, as Tom was helped, takes the edge off my sadness,' she concludes. 'This way, I can feel his presence all around me.'

Gunter L.

Shortly after Tom died, news reached me about a patient I had treated in Germany. I had been seeing Gunter L. over a period of years. Gunter also suffered from cancer. He was in his late fifties when we first met. Like Tom, he had gone through several periods of remission and relapse and was already in the late stages of his crippling illness. I taught him to use self-hypnosis as a general resource to provide meaning and purpose in what was left of his life; but, more specifically, for pain relief and to counteract the side-effects of his treatment.

When Leila, his wife, rang to tell me that Gunter had died, she mentioned something he had said shortly before he drifted into his final sleep. His message, apparently, was to thank me for the extra six years he believed I had given him.

What he said was: 'I'd have liked more, but I'll make do with what I have.' Leila and her family simply wanted me to know that, by using self-hypnosis in the way I had taught him, he managed to control his pain, and to die peacefully.

Mental attitude

Attitude of mind is a major part of the healing process in patients who have been diagnosed as suffering from any serious or life-threatening disease. Such an experience can wreak havoc with the emotions with the result that, when friendships are struck up among such patients, they tend to last. Some form groups among themselves, meeting frequently, to relax in each other's company.

One group of eight women (all of whom I have treated at some point in their illness) meets weekly for an informal get-together in a country pub. They have lunch and a chat, followed by an afternoon of leisurely activities. In the summer of 1996, when my wife was visiting South Wales, she was invited to join the friends at one of those lunches.

She thoroughly enjoyed their company, finding their attitude both encouraging and inspiring. 'Morbid' is the very last word she says she would use to describe this lively group.

'What's the point in being fatalistic?' reflected the most philosophical of their number.

Over a hearty meal, washed down by some pleasant wine, the friends shared family anecdotes, passed around photographs of children, grandchildren and pets: they talked about plans for Christmas, parties, holidays, the latest fashion trends and so on. It was all very relaxed and enjoyable. The selection of *risqué* jokes, from both sides of the table, helped remove the last vestiges of stress. Personally, I think this sort of social get-together is a great idea, and where better to have them than in the relaxed ambience of a pub?

Swapping anecdotes and memories, having a laugh: it is all good, clean fun and works a treat in terms of taking one's mind off one's troubles. Distractions and diversions such as these are the perfect antidote to stress; a state of mind which serves only to make matters worse. My wife's impression of the group she met for lunch was that, on the face of it they could have been members of a social club, an art-appreciation class, or simply business colleagues snatching a little time away from professional duties. Few would suspect all had been diagnosed as suffering from serious conditions.

Six were recovering from cancer surgery and coping with the aggressive drug therapy which normally follows such procedures. The other two were suffering from multiple sclerosis and clinical depression.

Those suffering from cancer reported that coping with their own fears was bad enough but, with mutual support and encouragement, they managed. The moments of light relief were particularly enjoyable, but also very necessary. What proved more difficult – despite all the publicity relating to health education in society these days – was the reaction of others.

'You wouldn't believe how many people still think they can "catch" the disease from us,' reflected one sufferer. 'We're quite used to being avoided once people know the nature of our illness.'

Her friend had a different theory about why former friends and acquaintances had begun to shun them.

'Couldn't it simply be that the whole idea embarrasses them so much they have to turn away?'

The observation sparked off something in the woman suffering from depression and she broke down into floods of tears. Through her sobs, she announced that her own illness was as nothing by comparison.

Then she apologized for upsetting them and believed her presence at future lunches to be inappropriate.

'I'm sorry,' she kept repeating. 'I shouldn't be here. I'm upsetting the rest of you.'

The others were appalled.

'You'll upset us a lot more if you don't come,' argued the woman sitting next to her. 'Don't you understand that your depression is an illness, just like ours? We feel for you. We relate to you.' She placed a protective arm around her friend. 'We don't want you to be lonely and miserable, because we're all here for each other.'

The love and support of those who cared about that woman helped ease her depression and reduce her stress until at last she was able to relax again and enjoy the congenial company.

It was precisely that sort of attitude and the emotional support it engendered that provided – and continues to provide – meaning and purpose in the lives of these eight friends. They were echoing my own belief in the importance of relieving anxiety and helping others cope with stress.

When life is not going too well for one of the cancer patients, it may turn out to be the woman suffering from depression who is called on to help.

Before leaving the topic of the pub lunch, I should add that these patients know that death may no longer be something remote, but they leave it aside at the lunch table nevertheless. Time enough to be serious later. When death occurs among those they have befriended, the process of bereavement hits hard. They have seen many go through the terminal stages of their illness. The relaxed atmosphere of those weekly lunches helps assuage the shock and numbness which invariably precede acceptance.

Children

Child care and development are never far from the minds of these women, particularly those not yet in their forties. Again, they are not being fatalistic, merely adopting a responsible attitude. The ongoing welfare of children is a matter to which all families struck down by serious illness should give some thought. Parents are not always aware of how their illness might affect academic and personal progress. During a recent seminar for teachers, patients showed how they coped as a family and how centres such as the Sandville could be of further benefit for their children. A small self-help group for eleven to sixteen-year-olds, begun in 1989, currently meets every month. Open to any child who has suffered the loss of a parent or sibling through bereavement or divorce, it is called RACEY: the initials standing for the Reassurance, Affection and Compassion it offers for Energetic Youths.

Children who have lost their parents suffer deeply, and the signs are not always interpreted correctly by those who take over their care. Behaviour problems are commonplace. These children can be disruptive in the classroom, school work can drop off, they frequently withdraw into themselves and suffer quietly alone. This is unfortunate because, in my experience, bereaved children respond well to hypnosis. As with adults, the greater the need for help, the faster the response.

Self-hypnosis can help them deal with whatever difficulties life in the absence of their parents might present. It can boost confidence, lower stress levels, help concentration at school and at home. It can remove the terror of impending exams.

Children can be treated from a relatively early age, virtually as soon as they have reached the use of reason. The only requirement for those who come to me for treatment is that they understand what they are being asked to do. This means that they need to be at least seven years old.

At the self-help centre, they attend in groups, because being in the company of those they know and trust makes the induction easier. Each young patient is treated on an individual basis. It is usually more satisfactory to see them in groups because, once they have witnessed the successful treatment of a friend or relative, any fear or apprehension they may have been harbouring about hypnosis vanishes. Then *they* can be treated with equal success.

To safeguard against any inherited tendency towards chronic or life-threatening illnesses, I suggest to the immune system that it should pay particular attention to attacking any cell malformations in order to restore the body's defences to normal.

Yes, it is a long term responsibility if the patients are very young but, to my mind, one which is well worthwhile.

When I treat children at home, it is always in the presence of a parent or guardian (and the family doctor if he wishes to join them). What do I treat them for? Bed-wetting, nail-biting, lack of confidence, exam nerves and all the usual problems from which children are likely to suffer, as well as any underlying illnesses, of course.

It has been proved time and again that, once a therapist understands the basics of how to reactivate the immune system, hypnosis can attack many disease states previously considered untreatable.

Notes
1 Information about testicular cancer can be obtained from the Imperial Cancer Research Fund, P.O. Box 123, Lincoln's Inn Fields, London WC2A 3PX.
2 The Sandville has its own registered School of Reflexology.

7   For Pain Relief

Self-hypnosis can be regarded as a treatment in its own right and as a valuable aid to more conventional forms of therapy. It is particularly beneficial as a means of pain relief, and the origin of the pain is irrelevant. Migraine, backache, arthritis, injuries resulting from sport and road traffic accidents have all been successfully treated in this way.

Natural warning system

When we are in trouble, pain acts as our natural warning system, and the beauty of hypnosis is that we can switch it off at source. The original message goes from the site of the wound or surgical incision to the brain; in blocking the pain response we can prevent the trouble at source. It is just as important to do this in the treatment of relatively minor conditions as it is in major disease. Pain and blood flow are both responses to the brain and the more we worry, the greater our pain and blood loss. Reduce the worry, and the rest follows automatically.

Patients undergoing dental surgery, women in labour and anyone else who might be expected to experience pain can be taught to control it before it has a chance to take hold. In cases of sudden unexpected bleeding, instructions can be given to the unconscious to constrict the relevant blood vessels.

Headaches

The cause of a headache can be a knock on the head, hunger, a hangover, sinus trouble, eye strain, toothache, lack of sleep; it can be the result of sitting in a noisy, stuffy, or smoke-filled room. If, after a full investigation, the doctor has eliminated all those possibilities and the diagnosis is migraine, the usual treatment is to prescribe some form of medication to be taken on a regular basis, although a few of my more enlightened medical friends have been known to suggest hypnosis.

They tell me that the only time to suspect an underlying problem is if the headache is accompanied by vomiting, slurred speech, difficulty in focusing, numbness in any part of the body, lack of concentration, loss of memory, confusion, high fever, or a stiff neck. In such cases, it is not hypnotherapy the sufferer needs, but urgent medical attention, because there is obviously something seriously wrong.

Migraine

Migraine is believed to afflict four million people in Britain every year. Most of the sufferers are women and one of the major factors triggering off the condition is stress. Migraine sufferers want fast relief from their pain, but removing the stress that caused the pain is equally important.

Jean P. was a typical migraine sufferer. She had, she explained, originally self-diagnosed her long-term headaches as emanating from a slowly developing malignant brain tumour. A highly imaginative type, Jean was given to nocturnal nightmares featuring near-death and out-of-body experiences. The prospect of surgery, radiotherapy, chemotherapy and possible insanity loomed large on her horizon. It never occurred to Jean that her condition could be anything less than terminal.

When she eventually plucked up the courage to visit her doctor, his diagnosis reassured her. He ruled out the possibility of serious illness and suggested she try hypnosis to relieve her anxiety.

Jean was a housewife and part-time secretary in her fifties. It is not her real name: I am respecting her wish for anonymity because, at the time of her referral, she had some domestic problems and asked not to be identified. When she telephoned me, early in 1997, she had been suffering from a series of what she described as 'blinding headaches'. What had once been occasional bouts of migraine had increased considerably in their frequency and were causing her great distress. An appointment was made for her and I suggested, as I invariably do, that she should bring along a trusted relative or friend.

In my experience, the patient always feels more relaxed in the company of someone who is close to them. In addition to that, as already explained, it makes the hypnotic induction easier to achieve. Jean and I met the following week, when she visited my home in the company of her daughter, Gill. She proved to be very responsive and, once relaxed, was taught how to use self-hypnosis.

The need to practise it regularly in order to achieve success was impressed upon her. The outcome of Jean's story is a happy one in several respects. Finding she could control subsequent attacks, she no longer needed to take prescribed medication. Her doctor was equally gratified that her long-standing migraine gave her no further trouble.

When she attended a few months later it was simply for a 'booster', because she felt a shade apprehensive about her imminent divorce and subsequent sale of the marital home. She had not actually had any further attacks of migraine, but the shadow of those awful headaches began to hover over her.

She was frightened that the upheaval in her domestic situation might stress her enough to provoke a fresh attack, if not a series of them. One does not need to be a migraine sufferer to feel the strain of a divorce and house sale.

The booster, or 'top-up' treatment was duly given, and once more Jean was ready to face up to her problems. In her most recent telephone call her voice sounded much more relaxed. She was living and working in a different part of the country and was happily involved in a new relationship. Best of all, she said, she had had no further attacks of migraine. As far as she was concerned, they had been consigned to history.

Learning to use self-hypnosis made a big impact on Jean's life. Her ability to remove headaches has been echoed many times over by others suffering from the same complaint; however, it is only fair to point out once more that migraine – like other conditions – can be treated only if its sufferers actually go under hypnosis, then practise self-treatment as advised, until it becomes habit.

Other forms of headache respond equally well to self-hypnosis. Doctors confirm what I have always believed: that most headaches are of simple origin and can be attributed to stress. Emotional stress, such as anxiety, depression or worry, can cause muscles to tighten and produce tension headaches. Hypnosis relieves pain and relaxes muscular tension. Stress overload is a problem in itself, but it can also cause, or contribute to, other health problems. The type of stress we build up every day varies from one type of personality to another, but the real problem is that we do not even know it is there until we exceed our tolerance level.

The effects of too much stress make themselves apparent in all kinds of ways. We know that stress and pain go hand in hand, with the result that millions of pounds are spent on pain-killers in the UK every year. All pain-killers are dangerous to the system, particularly those products containing aspirin and paracetamol. What makes them particularly hazardous is that they can be purchased over the counter (without a prescription) from supermarkets, corner shops, even garages, and people routinely devour them for headaches, hangovers and influenza.

To the delight of the pharmaceutical companies, who make huge profits from the sale of these drugs, an increasing number of them are now available without a prescription. What may not be generally known is how very few of these tablets it takes to reach overdose level, and how people vary in their susceptibility to the toxic effects.

Backache

Backache is another great problem in the western world and results in the loss of some thirteen million working days in Britain every year. More than half the population is believed to suffer from it at some time or other. The human spine is made up of twenty-four fragile bones which, with associated cartilage and tendons, support the entire weight of the upper body. Because the spine is such a complex structure and people do tend to overtax it, we should not be too surprised if things sometimes go wrong. The most common part of the back to be affected is down at the base of the spine, which is why people often say they are suffering from 'lower back pain'.

Back pain can come on suddenly and virtually incapacitate the sufferer. As with everything else, if it persists for more than a few days, it is advisable to pay a visit to the doctor to determine its possible cause. Gardening, lifting heavy loads, sitting uncomfortably, lying on a too-soft bed, overweight, or overexertion may be responsible. Whatever its cause, anxiety, stress and tension can make it worse. Some types of backache arise as a result of arthritis.

Arthritis

What exactly *is* arthritis? The word itself comes from the Greek (*arthron*, meaning joint; *itis*, meaning inflammation). It is so called because the main feature of the condition is inflammation, which, in turn, is due to some form of injury or damage. The pain of arthritis can be attributed to irritation of nerve endings within the affected joint or joints. In its most severe form, it can be a very debilitating condition.

Although we tend to think of arthritis as a condition primarily affecting the elderly, it can manifest itself at any age. While osteo-arthritis is more commonly seen in older people, rheumatoid arthritis can also affect infants and children. Osteo-arthritis is a degenerative disease affecting both sexes (in animals as well as humans). It is most common in people over the age of fifty and can affect virtually any joint in the body, whereas rheumatoid arthritis usually affects the hands and feet, producing swollen and tender joints which hurt when they are moved too much.

Arthritis can make the sufferer feel weak, tired and generally unwell. When it hits the spinal cord it can, quite literally, be a pain in the neck. Arthritis sometimes occurs on the site of an injury, or it can be associated with other conditions, the unsightly skin-scaling of psoriasis being one of them. Doctors usually prescribe anti-inflammatory tablets to reduce pain and swelling. While these tablets are intended to relieve the symptoms, they do not cure the underlying disease.

The best known anti-inflammatory is aspirin and the trouble with aspirin is that, when taken in the doses recommended for arthritis, its nasty side effects such as indigestion and stomach bleeding can be worse than the condition it is supposed to be treating. Milder drugs, with less dramatic side effects, are not much better. They all have the same effect on our body, that of rendering our own immune system redundant. Surely, it is better, if we know how to do it, to turn off the pain by natural means?

Ankylosing spondylitis

The strangely-named ankylosing spondylitis is another form of arthritis: in this case, stiffening of the bones in the spine. (Ankylosis is the consolidation of a joint; spondylitis is inflammation of the vertebrae).

Ankylosing spondylitis, therefore, is an inflammatory disease which causes the ligaments and bones of the spinal column to stiffen and become so rigid that they fuse together.

Terry C. wrote to me towards the end of 1996, having read my earlier book about the mind's ability to heal the body. 'You make a very positive case for the value of hypnosis in healing,' he stated. 'Having some problems with my neck, I visited the doctor and he diagnosed my condition as spondylitis. I feel sure you can help me to cope with it, through hypnosis.'

Terry added that he was particularly anxious not to have to rely on a regime of drugs, 'So please, may I have an early appointment?'

Naturally, I arranged to see Terry as soon as possible and am happy to report that he responded ideally both to the induction and to his lesson in self-hypnosis. I felt confident that this patient would practise daily to control his painful condition; which indeed, he did. Although I saw him on that one occasion only, he dropped me a line some three months later, to say that he was feeling fine.

So was this man's condition cured, or simply controlled? Who

knows? The fact that the chronic back pain and associated immobility no longer troubled him was all that mattered. Terry C.'s letter
carried a postscript saying that his doctor no longer felt the need
to prescribe any medication for him.

Marian Evans

Marian Evans, a former nursing sister, says she wishes she had
encountered hypnotherapy to help her patients in the hospital
where she spent many years as a busy theatre sister. Since her retirement in 1976, Marian always kept herself fit and active. She never
had any real physiological problems, apart from what she describes
as 'a touch of arthritis' following hip joint replacement surgery in
1983.

She was seventy-two years old when we met in August, 1988.

Here, in her own words, is what happened:

'You sat me down, and inducted me into a light state of hypnosis although, at the time I didn't realize that was what it was. The
treatment brought about an immediate improvement to my mobility, but something even more dramatic happened.

'I'd been on sleeping pills for twenty years. Suddenly, having
learned the technique of self-hypnosis, I knew I would never need
them again. It came as something of a shock to me as a nursing
sister; but I was determined to practise it every day, and I have done
precisely that.

'Self-hypnosis is proving ideal not just for insomnia and to
control general aches, but also for the purpose of eliminating stress.
I have used it to ease the pain of an inflammatory bladder condition, too.

'Hypnosis has calmed me down, stopped me worrying, helped
me relax. I just wish I had been familiar with this form of therapy
years ago. It should be included as a routine part of training for
nursing and medical students.'

Betty Barratt

Betty Barratt is another woman who swears by the therapeutic
value of hypnosis. A former community nurse, her activities in

retirement are mainly related to the Sandville Self Help Foundation, of which she is the current vice-chairperson.

Betty began to suffer from odd aches and stiffness in the joints of her hands and knees. She had watched me treat various patients and had a vague feeling that she too could benefit from my form of treatment, but felt others needed it more. Let Betty herself take up the story:

'One winter, during a particularly bad series of heavy snowfalls and gales, our telephone lines went down. Not being able to make or receive calls from the outside world, we never thought for one moment that you would be able to travel all the way down here from Merseyside. But you did, and there was only a handful of us here to greet you.

'Naturally, very few people turned up for the hypnotherapy session so I seized my moment, and took my turn for the "hot seat". I managed to enter a deep enough state to learn self-hypnosis and have been using it frequently ever since, practising it originally for several times a day, then twice a day for six months, and now, once a day, which is what I intend to do for the rest of my life. It's very beneficial, because I'm having no more pain in my hands and knees; I'm able to lead a normal life.

'All I can say, is thank God you came that day, because you haven't just taken away my pain, you've helped me with self-confidence, made me more energetic and brought about a general feeling of well-being. That's not bad, for someone aged seventy-one, is it?'

Yes, I must agree with Betty, it is not bad at all. But I did have to stress to her, to Marian and all the other patients who have had their mobility restored so satisfactorily that they must understand their own limitations.

While these energetic septuagenarians and others like them may feel they are twenty-one again, they are not, and should avoid running up and down stairs, or scaling ladders to decorate the house. Most senior citizens can compete mentally with their junior counterparts, but trying to compete physically is pure folly. Sports personalities and athletes are the first to admit that, once they reach early middle age, they must think in terms of a new career. The human body, like any machine, suffers from wear and tear and needs to be treated accordingly.

In my experience, most arthritic sufferers are a definite personality-type; the sort of people who spend their time bustling about, racing against the clock; in other words, attempting to do so much that they never allow themselves a minute to sit back and relax. My message to those who fall into that category is invariably to slow down. While they may have learned to remove pain almost instantaneously, they should appreciate that damaged joints take longer to heal and will do so only if they are not overtaxed.

Sometimes, when patients begin to feel better, they resume physical work and overindulge in the energetic pursuits. It is a great temptation, when free of pain, to catch up on the odd jobs which have been mounting up during the period of immobility. Then, hey presto, before they know what is happening, back comes the old familiar pain. That is the body's warning signal of impending trouble.

All of those patients whom I treat and teach self-hypnosis as a means of producing endorphins to combat pain have one important detail impressed upon their minds. It is that they are merely removing pain, not curing its cause.

They are clearly and frequently instructed that if the pain keeps returning, they must visit their doctor to find out why. Arthritis sufferers, once they have removed the pain of their condition, generally feel so good that they resume their erstwhile busy activities. When pain returns, it must be acknowledged as a warning to ease off on the activities. 'Stop what you are doing,' I tell them. 'Sit down and remove the pain in the manner taught. You must allow your body to heal itself, and to continue the healing process. If the pain is not to take hold once more, the brakes must be slammed on immediately.'

Strangely enough, the reverse situation also applies. Sometimes, when a patient's stiff limb is restored to mobility, it takes a while to grow accustomed to the fact that it can now move freely. The former sufferer continues to limp, even in the absence of pain in a knee, or hip joint. When limping has become a habit, it is difficult to break it.

Industrial and other injuries

John P. suffered from a painful shoulder following an industrial accident: a condition which had rendered his right arm virtually immobile. In time, his long-standing ache became aggravated by what his doctor diagnosed as spinal arthritis. The pains in his shoulder and back moved to his neck and he could hardly move without prescribed medication. He could not raise his arm at all.

John responded well to hypnosis; his arthritis and associated aches and pains were treated with successful results. He was, however, one of those frustrating individuals who refused to believe that he was actually under hypnosis because he was aware of everything going on around him. John claimed that, on arousal from what had, in fact, been a very deep state of hypnosis, his arm was still immobile. I casually asked how high he had been able to raise it before the accident. He demonstrated with a dramatic movement which lifted the arm high up over his head. His action surprised no one more than himself, and it finally convinced him that he had actually entered the necessary state of hypnosis.

A young woman called Sarah also took some convincing. Sarah had suffered extensive leg injuries following a road traffic accident some years before we met. Like John, Sarah responded readily to hypnosis and also had difficulty accepting that she had been in that state. Being able to walk without the arthritic pain which had set in on the site of her injuries seemed too good to be true. 'This can't be happening . . . I'm dreaming,' she insisted. 'I must be.' It was not until she awoke the following morning, with legs which were still free of pain, that she realized that she genuinely had been under hypnosis and that if she did not practise self-treatment, as taught, she would soon revert to her former state. We both knew of a patient who had been successfully treated for irritable bowel syndrome, but who did not practise self-hypnosis to keep the condition at bay. Predictably, it returned and brought with it a new problem: panic attacks.

I responded to that patient's request for further treatment because she sounded so distressed. This time, she promised herself daily treatment.

The problem which led Phoebe to my clinic in the autumn of 1997 had developed during the six months or so before her visit. Phoebe, a gifted young musician, had suddenly developed the very painful – and in her case thoroughly debilitating – condition known as repetitive strain injury (RSI). The condition, more frequently seen in newspaper reporters and others using computer keyboards hour after hour without a break, causes tendons in the wrists and arms to seize up, until excruciating pain results. Phoebe was a 'cellist and had been putting in long hours at her instrument in order to acquire the correct instrumental technique and all the other skills necessary to enable her to turn professional. As her condition worsened, her wrists stiffened so much she could hardly move them: in agony, she begged her doctor for pain relief.

Anti-inflammatories were prescribed and, despite taking them for some months, the 'cellist felt no better. After two or three minutes of daily practice, she was right back where she started. The pain and inflammation were as bad as ever. Another visit to the doctor resulted in referral to a specialist. The consultant assessed the situation and referred Phoebe to a physiotherapist.

'I was told I had developed muscle lesions from playing too much,' she explained. 'My posture was bad, and I wasn't taking enough rest between sessions. The physiotherapist gave me deep massage and we went through a series of exercises. She believed my condition was improving. If it was, there was no sign of it in my playing.'

The trouble was that Phoebe's unconscious mind did not accept what she had been told. Even after all the treatment, exercises and facing the prospect of improved posture, she still felt pain. Every time she picked up the bow and attempted to play her 'cello the pain returned and with it the inflammation. Her posture was no better either.

Phoebe responded readily to hypnosis and, as is customary with all my patients, was taught to put right the malfunctioning parts of her body, paying particular attention to the muscles, nerves and tendons in her arms and wrists. Then I taught her self-hypnosis, so that she could continue the process herself, by practising at least twice daily. I gave her a set of cards for self-treatment and suggested that, to sustain the success of her treatment, she should address the problem at its most basic level by telling herself: 'At the count of five, you, my unconscious mind will make me fully confident to play my 'cello, with no aches or pains. That is an order. One, two, three, four, five . . .' She should leave her UNS in no doubt as to who was boss. I assured her this type of instruction never failed.

The outcome of Phoebe's case was satisfactory. A few weeks later, *en route* to a chamber concert at which she was to perform that evening, our young 'cellist called in to see me. 'I read from your little cards every day,' she announced, 'and each time I put myself into hypnosis, I tell myself my wrists won't give me any more trouble. After that one treatment from you, the RSI hasn't bothered me at all, and I use the emergency count-to-five before every performance. That's never let me down, either.'

'It never will,' I assured her.

Phoebe needed no reminding that self-hypnosis must be practised every day for its beneficial effects to be felt. Nor did she need me to recapitulate that the 'customized cards' were also essential. Those who rely on their memory often find their abilities fading for the simple reason that they are not using the exact words as printed on the cards. The mental computer, like its man-made version, will only respond to instructions which have been fed in. If the words are not exactly right, it will fail to respond, as some patients have discovered to their cost.

8   For Stress Release

Stress

What *is* stress? As I see it, it is a blanket term covering many factors, chief among them being depression, worry, frustration, fear and grief. When stress develops beyond a certain point and becomes dangerous to the conscious, the unconscious begins to react, with the result that we start developing all those negative feelings. Stress is our body's response to the demands placed upon it. Going for an interview causes stress, so does taking a driving test. In each case, the reaction is the same: a quickening of the pulse, rapid breathing, and a general feeling of anxiety (young acne sufferers often find the trouble flaring up during end-of-term school exams). The concert pianist about to go on stage and the business executive preparing to give a presentation can also feel stress.

The difference is that those in the first group would describe the stress they feel as negative, whereas the second group might view it more positively. Actors, performers and others in the public eye frequently claim that stress is what gets them going, keeps them on their toes, makes them give of their best. That is all very well, provided they do not exceed their stress-tolerance level. Each one of us responds in our own particular way.

Some of us tolerate pain better than others and the same applies to stress. Stage and television personalities, business tycoons – even politicians – invariably have the type of personality that needs a stiff challenge to give them their 'high'.

Redundancy

In a situation where the challenge has gone and is replaced only by frustration at not being able to do anything worth while, the story is very different. Marie P. had worked for many years as practice manager for a team of busy dentists. Married to a bank manager, and the mother of two grown-up children, she enjoyed the stimulus of going to work, her status within the practice and she appreciated the independence her moderate salary allowed. The couple lived in a relatively affluent suburb of a northern city. Then, without warning, Marie's husband, Alan, was made redundant.

Their changed financial circumstances involved selling the large family house and moving to a bungalow some miles away: which, in turn, meant that Marie too was without a regular income. Worse still, she knew no one in the village where they now lived.

Alan, being a more phlegmatic type than Marie, settled into the new environment and life style without any great difficulty. But not Marie. She had enjoyed her work and the general buzz attached to the dental practice. An attractive, elegant woman, who was also a most efficient member of the team, she had been respected and admired by patients and colleagues alike. To have all of that suddenly taken away, through no fault of her own, proved a very great shock to her system.

Marie hated village life and had nothing in common with her new neighbours. She could not settle in the bungalow, but could see no way out. Feelings of hopelessness overwhelmed her: she lost interest in herself and allowed depression to take over.

She seldom arose before midday and when she did she slouched around in her housecoat, rarely venturing out of doors. Alan did his best to cheer her up. He suggested she should find herself a hobby, get out and about, visit their children, anything, to remove her self-inflicted stress. But it was hopeless.

Marie's stress became so severe that it produced a host of signs and symptoms, all of which arose from her negative attitude and overwhelming sense of loss. Would nothing lift her depression? She felt vulnerable and emotionally fragile. One part of her knew full well that stress was controlling her life, but another part associated the stress and depression with shame and it was that shame which prevented her from seeking help.

Alan could not force her to. Deep down, he sensed that, unless his wife 'bucked up her ideas' (his words), he would lose her altogether. And lose her, he did. At the age of fifty-two, Marie had a cerebral haemorrhage (stroke) and died.

The death certificate gave the cause of death as atheroma (hardening of the arteries), but in real terms, it was boredom, causing stress. I learned of Marie's case from Alan who approached me a year or so later asking if my form of treatment could help him cope with his grief. I am delighted to say that it did. It also gave him confidence in his own abilities; so much so that at the age of fifty-four he surprised everyone by applying for and obtaining a new post as financial adviser to a company that was setting up a branch near his new home. The work was nothing like as high-powered as that at the bank, but it gave him back his self-respect and his motivation to go on.

The message coming through from this salutary tale is that when people are in control, they can deal with anything life throws at them; when they are overstressed, they can deal with next to nothing. If the power of the mind over the body is remarkable, that of the unconscious over the conscious is even more so.

Bernard F. was an auditor who, like Alan, was in his early fifties, had recently been made redundant and did not feel ready for retirement. In common with most men in middle management, Bernard had been given a reasonable pay-off and wanted to put it to good use. He had set his heart on purchasing an antiquarian bookshop. Contracts had been drawn up (but not yet exchanged) and all systems were go. Then, unexpectedly and for no apparent reason, Bernard began to feel uneasy. His intention in requesting hypnotherapy was for the purpose of relaxation. He was on the brink of embarking on a new career, he told me, and he wanted to be more laid back about it.

Bernard's response to hypnosis was excellent and during the course of treatment I gave him access to his unconscious memory, as I do to all my patients. This meant that he could, if he wished, bring back all the emotional, physical and sensual aspects of any given incident in his life. Instructed to allow his memory to drift back to the cause of his stress, he did precisely that. Deep in hypnosis, the brows of his still-closed eyes rose as if seeing again something which alarmed him:

'Bloody hell!' he exclaimed. 'How could I have missed that?'

'Missed what?' I asked.

'The discrepancies . . . the accounts books have been completely falsified.'

I left him to conduct a mental re-examination of the ledgers for a few moments in silence, then returned him to the present and aroused him from hypnosis. The cause of Bernard's stress was now patently clear to him. The mystery had been solved.

But why should he have reacted in this way?

Easy. He had wanted to buy the bookshop so much that the dodgy paperwork had been deliberately overlooked by his conscious mind, but the 'watchman' inside him, his unconscious, was having none of it. The UNS overlooks *nothing*. Hence the conflict . . . and the stress. Having uncovered the cause of his stress, Bernard was able to dispose of it.

Needless to say, he did not buy the bookshop. When I last met him he was doing the rounds of estate agencies to see what else was on offer. The case of Bernard and the shop purchase that never was might not seem to have been very serious in terms of the man's health. Yet there is no doubt that it would have been had it been allowed to get out of hand. Troubles arising from the purchase of that propery, had it gone ahead, would not have been confined to the financial.

We should never underestimate the seriousness of stress. It is one of the world's greatest killers, contributing to coronary and arterial disease, cancer and a wide range of other illnesses. Many factors can be responsible, ranging from overwork to emotional disturbance, difficult living conditions and unhappy personal relationships.

Currently, the damaging effects of stress are believed to cause more than ninety million working days to be lost in Britain every year. In a survey conducted by The Institute of Management, 50 per cent of the country's employees agreed that they did not look forward to going to work.[1]

Bereavement

Learning self-hypnosis is the ideal means of teaching people to rid themselves of stress and all its connotations. Richard Grebham, a 23-year-old theology student is one young man who has benefited considerably from the technique. The circumstances under which we first met were somewhat traumatic, in that he (like Alan, the former bank manager whose story is recounted above) had been recently bereaved.

'My mother had just died of cancer,' he recalls 'and I was stressed-out. You were talking to a group of people about what could be achieved through hypnosis and I sat at the back of the room listening to your words. I was intrigued, and immediately volunteered to try out the technique. Before I realized it, I felt myself slipping into hypnosis.'

Richard practises regularly and sees me for 'top-up' treatments to help with revision for his exams.

'Before learning the technique of self-hypnosis, my problem was that I couldn't finish the papers in the allotted time. Afterwards, the difference immediately became apparent. The very next time I had to face an exam, I put myself into hypnosis before going into the room and told myself I would have no further trouble.

'It worked fine. I raced through the papers with confidence. I know now that they will never be a problem again . . . all because you instructed me to tell my unconscious to use *its* memories to help with my studies. So that's what I've been doing, and it's been great.'

Richard came on so well during the following academic term that he found himself far enough ahead to take a year out from his studies to do something else he had wanted to do for some time: work in bar-management. As a future minister of religion, he believed that type of administration would give him a deeper insight into human nature!

Pressures of work

Stress is today's buzz word. Whether we like it or not, it is constantly there, in the background of our lives, lurking in the undergrowth, like a big cat waiting to pounce. Doctors, nurses, journalists and business executives are the first to admit that the pressures of their work put them constantly under stress. But how many people actually admit to suffering from it? Like the ill-fated Marie, who refused to seek help, they believe stress has connotations of weakness and failure.

People who are over their stress tolerance level do not think or act rationally. They convince themselves they can cope, or have a vague feeling that perhaps they will be able to cope when the circumstances causing their stress are changed. That is not necessarily so. Complete removal of stress is achieved by unconscious mechanisms only.

While yoga, meditation and the like do help during the actual period of treatment, their effects soon wear off and sufferers frequently find themselves back where they started, because fundamentally they do not penetrate the mind in the way that self-hypnosis does.

Yoga – which is incorporated into Hindu religious philosophy – aims to merge the human spirit with that of the universe. Hatha yoga (the type most commonly practised in the West) is a system of posture and breathing exercises intended to relieve stress and improve general health. Meditation concentrates on attempts to achieve a higher state of consciousness. It does so by use of a mantra (word, or series of words) in order to achieve inner-awareness. Meditation uses imaginative processes to induce a state of calm and well-being, in order to bring peace of mind.

There is a move in some of our larger teaching hospitals for medical and nursing staff to be given counselling at the end of particularly difficult days on the ward or in the theatre to prevent them taking their stress home. This is an excellent idea because there must surely be few situations more stressful in one's daily life than constantly having to face the sick and dying. Small wonder that the suicide rate is so high among these professionals and that so many doctors and nurses turn to alcohol.

With journalists and business executives, the circumstances are rather different. On the whole, these highly motivated professionals only function efficiently with deadlines and multimillion corporate decisions looming.

Journalists and business executives are competitive people, and competitive people thrive on being supercharged. Like athletes and racing drivers, they feel that, once their systems are fired and the adrenalin has begun to pump, they can go anywhere, do anything. Creative people *need* these bursts of energy to produce their best results. When they fall into the trap of alcoholism, it is more likely to be the result of too many expense account lunches than the fear of being unable to cope. One must be careful not to confuse stress with challenge.

Overindulgence in food, drink and physical exertion are no good for anyone, but then, how much is too much? The boundaries between healthy pressure and unhealthy stress are not easily defined and whereas one individual can stand up to all sorts of pressures, another can crack at the slightest strain. I spend half my life telling people there is no shame attached to being stressed.

Stress creeps up on individuals, sometimes without any warning. As with the proverbial camel, it was not the load that broke the unfortunate animal's back, it was the addition of that one extra straw. With us it is often that one final 'straw' which does the damage. There is only so much stress anyone can take. Inanimate objects are similarly affected. The slender rope that ties a rowing-boat to a pier, the huge steel hawser that ties up the ocean liner, both will break if stressed beyond their limit.

Drinking to excess
Flying would never be my chosen means of transport; I would always opt for the more leisurely pace of overland or sea travel. It has nothing to do with fear.

I simply prefer one to the other, in the same way that I prefer a hot meal to a salad, detective television programmes to soap operas.

When I heard what Colin P. had to tell me, I was even less enamoured of the prospect of air travel.

Colin was a senior captain flying jumbo jets for an international carrier based in the United States. He had coped admirably with his duties for twenty years or more; but now, increasing demands were being made on him. The arrival of younger, fitter colleagues had never been a problem and probably still would not be, he confessed, had the situation not been compounded by pressures building up at home. His marriage was going through a rough patch, his daughter was about to leave home and marry. Expenses attached to the wedding were rocketing and Colin was sinking deeper and deeper into debt.

He was drinking too much and sleeping too little, thus endangering the lives of hundreds of passengers every time he took control of his aircraft. He was due for a medical soon and was very worried at the prospect of being grounded and frankly, noticing the restlessness and high anxiety state of a man I imagined to have once been calm and easy-going, I could not see any other outcome. I was surprised only that he had held his post for so long. Colin was overweight, out of sorts and looked like a four-ulcer man in a five-ulcer job.

And yes . . . he did go under hypnosis, he did succeed in learning self-treatment and he did practise it on a regular basis. But no, he did not pass his medical; nor did I expect him to. Quite apart from the fact that his fondness for drink had not gone unnoticed by his superiors, he was no longer in his prime.

Self-hypnosis can achieve remarkable effects, but it cannot perform miracles.

I heard no more from Colin until the invitation to his daughter's wedding dropped on my doormat. Curious as to his fate, I accepted. If seeing the change in his general health and demeanour surprised me, the surprise was nothing compared with that on discovering that not a drop of alcohol passed his lips all day. Over a quiet glass of apple juice, Colin explained that on his enforced retirement, he had put his cards on the table; first to his own family, then to the family of his prospective son-in-law. As a result, the groom (who, as a computer consultant, was earning a respectable salary) had agreed to share the expenses of the wedding. So that was one worry off Colin's mind.

The prospect of endless empty days ahead was resolved in a rather different way. Colin took himself to an animal rescue centre and adopted the largest, most energetic dog in their kennels. His new friend Bouncer kept him on his toes and ensured that he had plenty of physical exercise. The stress had gone from Colin's life and his marriage difficulties had been resolved. He was practising self-hypnosis regularly and everything in the garden was lovely.

Colin had not actually been an alcoholic, but during his period of severe stress, he had been in very real danger of becoming one. The question thus arises as to whether hypnosis might have helped him, if he *had* been an alcoholic.

I must be honest. In my experience, with alcoholism and smoking, the success rate is small because no hypnotist can make people do what they do not want to.

Those who approach me asking for help to stop drinking, or smoking, might claim they want to give up the habit; but deep down, this is seldom strictly true. Because of his own determination, and for no other reason, Colin might have been helped if he had gone over the borderline into addiction. As it was, self-hypnosis gave him the extra incentive he so desperately needed. Once he had control over his unconscious mind, because he genuinely wanted to stop drinking, he was taught to treat himself.

While drink and cigarettes may appear to relieve anxiety, the effect, like that produced by meditation or yoga is limited, and soon wears off with the result that the craving may well increase. In other words, when the effect wears off, the stress is even greater than before. During hypnosis, as during sleep, we repair and renew ourselves to wake up invigorated. A few minutes of self-induced hypnosis can achieve the same effect as a whole night's sleep.

Drinking and smoking are common stress-relievers. Hypnosis can reduce or stop the intake, but without learning the technique for removal of stress, the habit, or addiction, invariably returns. Hypnosis is ineffective in terms of stopping people smoking or drinking, but those who are so inclined can be enabled to stop these practices themselves. The same applies to over- (or under-) eating.

Food can be a great solace or it can be a dramatic form of self-punishment in cases of guilt. The subject of guilt is so vast and complicated that it will be studied independently in a later chapter. In my experience, only occasionally do people suffering from eating disorders respond to hypnosis.

The reason is that most of them do not accept that they have any need of treatment. The few patients who have responded have done so because they were aware of the existence of some underlying problem (though not of its nature) which needed to be rooted out and disposed of first.

Colin was an extrovert, but more introspective types also have their problems. Put a quiet, sensitive, person into a work situation where everyone else is noisy and aggressive and that person will soon begin to feel the strain; likewise a noisy extrovert restrained within the confines of somewhere like a reference library, or a monastery.

Frightening situations

Fear, as we have seen, causes various changes to occur in the body: our breathing becomes shallow, our heart thumps, mouth dries up, palms perspire, shivers run up and down our spine. Just picture the situation. You are on a pedestrian crossing as a car approaches at speed. Will the driver stop in time? Or perhaps you are at home, alone. In the middle of the night, a brick comes flying through the bedroom window and, suddenly, heavy footsteps cross the room. Is the intruder armed? While it is perfectly understandable to panic at times like this, the question might arise as to why these sorts of situation should provoke the type of response they do?

The answer is that because, deep down, fear is something else we have inherited from our prehistoric ancestors. We are echoing what went on millions of years ago when primitive man had to prepare himself for danger. It is what is known as the fight-or-flight response: Nature's way of protecting us.

Faced with imminent danger, our body reacts in the same way as his. Should we fight or flee? The very idea puts us into a state of anxiety and the resulting stress activates our aches and pains. It decreases the efficiency of our immune system. Flashing back through evolution, surely the most stressful event in any animal's life was the fear of being killed. Those who could fight the predator did so.

Coping with stress

Introverts may give an impression of being calm and laid back. But again, beneath the surface the introvert may be oversensitive and unable to cope with life's pressures. Only by accessing the unconscious is it possible to determine whether nature or unhappiness has produced the introvert's behaviour patterns.

In other words, when we start digging down to the root of the problem, do we uncover stress spreading its nasty tentacles throughout the undergrowth?

Note
1 Charlesworth, Karen, 'Are managers under stress?' A survey of management morale, published by the Institute of Management, London, 1996.

9   Other Problems

Lack of confidence

Dawn L. was a beautiful doe-eyed brunette, who had worked for many years as owner/proprietor of a flourishing fashion boutique but, thanks to the recession, her shop had had to close and Dawn was now unemployed. She came to my clinic with three related problems: lowered self-esteem now that she was no longer in business, fear that she would never work again, and a return of the asthma which had plagued her childhood. The asthmatic attacks had been increasing both in freqency and intensity since Dawn had been forced to shut up shop.

Dawn, in her white silk suit with diaphanous multicoloured scarf draped about her neck was quite the most elegant woman ever to have consulted me. She was also one of the most insecure. With looks like that, self-confidence should have been oozing from every pore, instead of which she was throwing out messages of gloom and despondency. I felt her tension as soon as she entered the room.

'There is nothing down for me,' came the opening gambit. The voice was shaky and tearful. She repeated the words several times during our consultation period. 'Nobody wants to employ a shop-keeper past her prime.'

It was a ridiculous claim. Dawn was certainly not past her prime. A quick assessment told me that her low self-esteem and belief in being unemployable had to be tackled first. With them out of the way, the asthmatic attacks would cease automatically. These attacks had, after all, arisen (as they had in childhood) because

Dawn acknowledged that while she was certainly not stupid, she was no mastermind. She was simply, to quote her own description, 'stressed up to the eyeballs', and I had to agree.

I made the point to Dawn, as I do to all my patients, that academic achievements and intelligence do not necessarily go hand in hand and the fact that she had left school without certificates was certainly not proof of an inferior brain. Indeed, the speed with which she entered hypnosis showed how intelligent she actually was.

Speaking directly to her unconscious, I instructed Dawn to put right whatever sections of her body were causing the asthmatic attacks, then I boosted her self-confidence and taught her how to reactivate the part of her personality which had given her the confidence to run her popular boutique in the first place.

'You must never again doubt your own abilities,' I told her. 'Find something new,' I suggested. 'You have reached a turning point in your life. You must channel your energies and undoubted talents in another direction. Find a new outlet for your skills. You can do it. You *must* do it,' I insisted.

Thinking a spot of 'smile therapy' might not go amiss, I asked her to tell her unconscious that she needed to laugh. Within minutes, she was laughing heartily. Stress-reduction takes many forms. The outcome of Dawn's story is that, following her treatment, she no longer views herself in such a negative light. As a result, there have been no further asthmatic attacks and, with her doctor's blessing, she has dispensed with her nebulizer and other prescribed medications.

The restoration of her self-confidence and renewed belief in herself meant that she was able to put her life back on track. Despite her age (which she never disclosed, but I guessed to be somewhere between forty and fifty), she was able to resume her career in the world of fashion retailing, albeit at first on a voluntary basis. She was, she told me with considerable enthusiasm, spending two days a week behind the counter of an 'upmarket' charity shop. The irony of the situation was that the shop was housed in the very unit that her own boutique had been. 'It's home from home, really,' she remarked.

Not only that, it had led to other opportunities. Dawn had given so many customers the benefit of her expertise in terms of how to wear their purchases with panache that word of her talents spread and groups of women were inviting her to come and show *them* how to make the best of themselves, by 'editing' their wardrobes on a fee-paying basis. She was soon earning more than she ever did in her boutique. To put it all on a professional basis, she took a part-time college course to train as an image consultant. Now with a certificate to her name, she could boost her funds even further. She was her own boss again, and loving every minute of it.

Speech impediments

There is an old saying that people who keep horses eventually begin to resemble them. In the same way, someone who shares a home with a partner or parent afflicted with a speech impediment is liable to end up with the same impediment. This is a concept I find myself having to bear in mind when approached by patients who have difficulty in making themselves understood. As Sherlock Holmes might have said, it is important to eliminate the simple solution, before seeking out the more complicated.

Children are renowned for copying their elders and it is not unknown for them to pick up hesitant speech patterns of parents just as they might pick up their regional accents. The easy way to determine whether this is what has happened is to establish whether a family member is (or ever was) so afflicted.

If not, then regression to the patient's formative years should produce results. More usually though, the faltering, repetitive words of the stammerer, the involuntary hesitation of the stutterer are due to stress. The stress in these situations is invariably associated with lack of confidence, which may well have originated *outside* the home. The repercussions of faulty teaching in the infant and junior school can manifest themselves far into adulthood.

Of course, I appreciate that teachers have a difficult job to do and my heart goes out to those in charge of unruly adolescents. No one would dispute that their work is difficult and stressful and I am always happy to co-operate with education authorities who invite me to address groups of teachers and lecturers on the subject of stress control.

Many of those who attend these lectures realize that they do have a problem and subsequently request treatment on an individual basis; follow-up enquiries show that they have been able to cope much better in their classrooms and lecture halls as a result. One of the messages I try to impart to educators is about the influence – good and bad – they have on young minds. Intentionally or otherwise, teachers can make a deep impression on children; so deep, in fact, that it can affect them for decades ahead.

A teacher, faced with a misbehaving child, should deal with that child firmly, but compassionately. Ideally, he (or she) should take the child to one side and reprimand it quietly.

With older sufferers, there is another possibility. Teachers of earlier generations believed there was something inherently wrong with a child who was left-handed and they routinely tried to get that child to write with the right – the 'correct' – hand. This often involved tying the offending hand behind the back. The teacher would then order the child to use the right hand, and would supervise the often tearful attempts.

The confidence of these children was so shattered that some reacted to the enforced change of what they considered to be normal behaviour by developing speech impediments. Others reverted to bed-wetting, or even thumb-sucking. Thankfully, left-handedness is no longer a stigma.

Teachers should inspire confidence and individuality in their charges, not suppress them. They should address themselves to the business of teaching, without allowing their own stresses to overflow into vindictiveness. They should motivate the children in their care, not devalue them.

Starting school is usually the first occasion on which a child leaves its mother and home. Children do not always have the ability to cope with strange people in a strange environment. Unsympathetic teachers are the last thing they need.

The words and actions of teachers can have a very far-reaching effect, indeed.

Cross-dressing

Gareth L.'s problem was, admittedly, not of the type one encounters every day. His reason for approaching me was that he was a transvestite: he liked to dress up in women's clothes. Unlike some cross-dressers he was not behaving in that way because he enjoyed the feel of women's clothes on his body, but because of an inexplicable urge within him. Otherwise, he was perfectly normal in every respect and earning a good living as a civil servant (in conventional suit, collar and tie which, incidentally, was his mode of dress when he came for therapy).

However, as soon as he arrived home each evening, Gareth donned the garments of the person he liked to think of as Gloria. He had no desire to *be* a woman, just to *dress* like one. Could he find out, through hypnosis, why this should be? It was an unusual case; the only one of its type I had so far encountered, though I have since been given to understand that the general reason why men dress as women and – less frequently – women as men, is for stress-release. Instead of smoking, drinking or nail-biting, they 'step out of themselves' and adopt another persona. But not Gareth. His reason for cross-dressing turned out to have been the result of a traumatic experience in childhood.

Gareth had been an angelic-faced cherub with a mop of bubbly blond curls. Those who did not know him often thought he was a girl which, of itself, did not unduly bother the boy, until one day at school a particularly unpleasant teacher began to make fun of him. For reasons best known to herself she ridiculed Gareth and told him that as he looked so much like a little girl perhaps he had better be taught girls' subjects.

When, therefore, at the school's prize-giving ceremony the unfortunate Gareth was presented with a book about dressmaking he became an object of fun for the entire school. While the other boys were proudly showing off their carpentry tools and chemistry sets, Gareth was hiding away in a corner. Alone. He was not to know that the general derision he suffered thanks to that teacher's action would fester away in his mind for many years to come. Thankfully, it no longer does, but that teacher, wherever she is, has a lot to answer for.

Gareth's games master was no better than his insensitive female colleague. He ridiculed the boy because of his lack of sporting prowess. Ignoring objections and pleas to be excused, the teacher forced Gareth to play rugby and cricket, then howled with laughter at his pathetic attempts not to disgrace his team. Presumably it was the teacher's way of trying to toughen Gareth and turn him into something he was not. Left to his own resources this boy would have been much happier spending his leisure time indoors, strumming away at his guitar or reading a book – any book – except, maybe, the one on dressmaking!

Difficulty in forming relationships

In the normal run of events children are born with various talents and qualities. Some, like Gareth, are overendowed with beauty and sensitive creativity, while others appear to have been totally overlooked. Anyone who had ever encountered Matt C. would have to acknowledge that he was no oil-painting. A big, powerful man, he was chunky, fat, and gave the impression he could be handy with his heavily-tattooed fists. He looked like a boxer, although he was in fact a 'bouncer' at a prominent night club. Matt's powers of comprehension were a little on the slow side, but once the message penetrated he was fine.

This man was not unintelligent nor was he without certain skills, having recently completed a demanding course to train as a dog-handler. Why was it, he wondered, that he could relate so easily to animals but hardly at all to humans? He had never been popular, he went on to explain, even as a child. Where it had all started he had no idea, but then no one ever has any *conscious* idea of what might be causing their severe lack of confidence.

In Matt's case it was so deeply damaging that it took several sessions of therapy before I could get anywhere near the root of the problem. At last, under regressive hypnosis, it emerged that Matt's problem, like Gareth's, had originated in the classroom. Matt, being larger and fatter than his contemporaries, looked older, yet despite his size he was considerably less able to cope with the academic demands being made on him. To compound his problem, he too was hopeless at games.

As boys do, his classmates teased and bullied him mercilessly and his teachers were even worse. His form teacher accused him of being a stupid, fat fool and did not reprimand those who called him Fat Matt. All of that would have been enough to shatter anyone's confidence for life. I felt intensely sorry for Matt. Even after locating and apparently disposing of the problem, this man still needed a couple of further sessions to reinforce the message. It was necessary for me to repeat again and again that the jeerings to which he had been subjected were not only out of order, but also inaccurate. While we both agreed that he *was* seriously overweight he took some convincing that he was neither stupid nor a fool. Would the dogs he handled so competently have responded to him otherwise?

It was vitally important for Matt's health that the confidence he displayed with those dogs be reflected in his attitude to people. And ultimately it was. Patient and understanding teachers could have helped Matt through his difficulties instead of exacerbating them. I have lost count of the number of patients I have treated whose problems originated at school.

Lack of confidence causes so many intelligent children to fail their exams. Parents and siblings can also do considerable damage to formative young minds, as we shall see. Not only that, some of us manage to do it all by ourselves.

Motorway terror

The technique of regressive hypnotherapy will be fully explored in a later chapter but, while still on the subject of restoring confidence, let me relate the tale of Marianne T., a middle-aged housewife whose problem revolved around motorway driving. Marianne was an experienced driver who had never – to her knowledge – experienced any difficulties at the wheel in the thirty or so years since she had passed her test. But one day, out of the blue, she found she could not even entertain the idea of driving on a motorway. She went cold at the very idea. 'I wouldn't mind,' she sighed, 'but I've no knowledge of ever having had an accident, or even a near miss. So why am I freaking out like this? Where's my confidence gone? And, for pity's sake, why? Help, please. . . .'

Under hypnosis I suggested to her unconscious that she let her memory drift back to whatever the incident was which caused her sudden lack of confidence. And there she was, in a brand new vehicle, pulling out into the fast lane to overtake the slow-moving lorry in front; only when she pressed down on the accelerator, to her horror the car did not move swiftly forward as it should.

In that split second, Marianne's mind registered that she could not return to the middle lane, and the vehicle tailing her was too close to allow her to drop back.

Various thoughts raced through her mind: they came in microseconds and added up to one word: *danger*. Marianne's inner panic was so strong that her unconscious mind, sensing danger, blocked off the entire episode and refused to allow her to remember what happened next. In the belief that it was further protecting her, it also did its utmost to prevent her ever again driving on a motorway.

Now that she was in a position to recall what actually did happen, Marianne recalled how the vehicle, almost immediately and again of its own accord, picked up speed. She was safely in control once more. My role as therapist was to make this patient understand that her mental block had not been caused by any fault of her own, but by some technical 'blip' in the vehicle. That particular session of therapy was conducted in the company of several other patients, some of whom had already been treated, while others were still waiting. Among the group was a long-distance lorry driver, whom I had noticed nodding his head in the affirmative throughout Marianne's brief regression to her period of trauma. The moment her memories were returned to the present and she was aroused from hypnosis, he stepped forward to announce that it was a problem with which he was all too familiar.

'I've seen that sort of thing happen, myself,' he stated. 'A temporary block in the petrol feed can cause a vehicle to stall in exactly the way you described. It takes less than a minute, but it scares the hell out of you while it's happening. It always clears itself though.'

Motor vehicles generally

Francine's problem also related to driving, though in her case, it was not just motorways that scared her. When it came to taking control of the wheel, Francine displayed a total loss of confidence. In fact, she had not even taken her test and suspected she never would, being content to settle for taxis and public transport, making excuses that there were enough cars on the road and she was managing perfectly well without one.

Directed back to the cause of the trouble, this woman's memories came to an abrupt halt in the middle of a driving lesson. Her instructor had only that day shown her how to do an emergency stop when, suddenly, a small boy had jumped out from behind a hedge to retrieve a ball which had rolled directly into the path of the car. Within minutes of learning the procedure, Francine was having to do it for real.

She rammed both feet down, pressing brake and clutch pedal hard to the floor and managed to stop the vehicle within inches of the terrified child. No one was hurt in the incident, but Francine's shock at what had occurred shook her rigid. Her instructor congratulated her warmly on her swift action, told her she had displayed great presence of mind and praised the skilful way in which she had risen to the challenge of turning theory into practice.

He did not mind admitting that for a split second he too had experienced sheer terror at the thought of how a less competent driver might have reacted. Francine would have no difficulty in passing her test, he insisted. But this learner-driver was not convinced.

In spite of all her instructor's attempts to get her to resume the lesson, she insisted on swapping places and begged to be driven home. She never took the wheel again. Her self-confidence restored, under hypnosis, Francine thought she could now face the prospect of more lessons. To have a car of her own, she agreed, would enable her to get out and about much more than she did at present.

Socializing with peers

Hayley's family lived in a small semi-detached house in the suburbs of a West Country city. Her father, Bill, worked as a joiner, her mother, Vera, was a secretary by day, a barmaid in the evenings. Hayley was their only child. The family had no car and could not afford foreign holidays. Every penny they could spare was put aside to pay for their daughter's private education. Bill and Vera were determined to give Hayley the sort of opportunities they never had.

Hayley loved her parents dearly and was very grateful for their efforts, but would have much preferred to attend the local comprehensive school with her friends. She felt uncomfortable and embarrassed at being educated alongside children whose parents were considerably richer than her own.

How could she possibly socialize with girls who boasted about their huge houses with swimming-pools and games-rooms? Hayley knew that most of the parents were professional people; she had seen them dropping off their daughters in top-of-the-range motor-cars. They wore expensive clothes and took their children – Hayley's classmates – on holiday two or three times a year, often to far-flung places she had never heard of.

Hayley did not resent their good fortune, but she did feel uneasy in their company. She could not accept their party invitations because she would be expected to return the compliment and that would embarrass her parents. She could not join their tennis club, or move in the same social set.

Nor could she mix any more with her former friends who were now moving in different circles. She even began to feel tense in the company of her parents. Through no fault of her own poor Hayley was as much a square peg at home as she was at school.

When she was eighteen years old, Hayley was brought to my clinic by her worried parents. A bungled suicide attempt had been, as they so often are, a 'cry for help'. After a brief spell in hospital, the girl seemed fine, but had totally lost her confidence. Bill's and Vera's deep concern was surpassed only by Hayley's own. My main regret in this case was that she had not come for treatment earlier.

Having learned self-hypnosis, Hayley was able to cope, for the first time in her life, with whatever the world had to throw at her. I feel it necessary to point out here that while I do not share the views of those who would deny parents the right to educate their children in whatever way they deem best, I do think that in this case, Hayley would have been better equipped to cope with life at the comprehensive school.

She would have enjoyed herself more in the company of classmates with whom she was already familiar, while Bill and Vera could have relaxed and enjoyed themselves without putting in such long hours and being constantly worried about school fees, uniform, text books and the like for their unhappy daughter.

Now this may seem like a complicated case, but it was not really. Hayley's confidence needed boosting. That was all. Her parents had done their best for her and she for them. It was only when the submerged feelings of self-doubt had begun to surface that the mental bubble had burst and she had swallowed enough paracetamol to raise the alarm but thankfully, not enough to kill her. Had she responded with tears or anger, and got the problem out of her system when her parents first suggested private education, it might not have caused such damage.

PART FOUR

Digging Deep into the Mind

10   Depression

More than half the patients who come to me for treatment are suffering from depression. Even among those who are not currently suffering from it, many have experienced depression at some stage in their lives. When that state of mind has continued over long periods and is so severe that it is affecting everyday functioning the patient needs professional help.

Depression makes people sad and pessimistic, leaving them with little interest in their surroundings. The reasons for their depression are as varied as the symptoms themselves. While it is natural to feel depressed because a close relative or friend has died, if depression occurs without obvious cause and worsens to the point when behaviour and health are affected, it is serious. Where there is an obvious reason for the depression, it is less so. Both types of depression can be treated by self-hypnosis. It is not surprising that some women become depressed on finding themselves pregnant for the first time. A mother-to-be, whose own mother died when she herself was a child, may feel uneasy about the concept of motherhood and all it entails, particularly if she has no elder sister or other knowledgeable relative to turn to for advice. Through self-hypnosis, such a patient can be taught to rely on her own judgement and to cope with each day as it comes.

In the same way, a person who has been recently bereaved can use self-hypnosis to facilitate adjustment to the grief. If the person who died was a partner, my custom is to ask whether the marriage, or relationship, was a good one. If so, then it helps if the bereaved person can be made to understand that the deceased person would hardly want those left behind to spend the rest of their days grieving in the manner of Queen Victoria for Prince Albert.

Types of depression

Fundamentally, there are two types of depression: reactive, which happens when the patient reacts to a particular event or series of events, and endogenous, which originates from deep inside.

Reactive depression sets in as a result of something like a bereavement, redundancy, bankruptcy, or other personal trauma which outsiders are prepared to accept as reasonable. The cause is obvious and the sufferer can remember all the details. Someone sitting at home without money or friends has good cause to be depressed. When circumstances improve the depression lifts.

Depression arising from known causes is also occasionally referred to as 'exogenous'; it describes people who are depressed because of a whole series of disasters (which they can recall). The words exogenous and endogenous have opposite meanings; the prefix 'exo' (of Greek origin) referring to external factors, 'endo' (also from the Greek) to those originating from within.

Endogenous depression is the most problematic to deal with because it is hidden far beneath the surface. People who endure this type of depression may think they know the cause of their problem but in fact the memories are so deep that they have no idea at all. This type has a sneaky habit of coming over the patient at any time and for no obvious reason.

In my experience, endogenous depression is *always* related to past trauma. To remove the trauma in its entirety therapeutic regression is called for.

Individual cases (Sheena, Leah, Simon)

Sheena had come to see me because she wanted to regress in the hope that recovery of a lost memory might be helpful to her. A young mother of three, she mentioned that she suffered from spasmodic attacks of depression for no apparent reason. Questioned about her childhood, she told me it was very happy and completely problem-free. She asked me to direct her memories back to a time before she was born. Sheena never suspected for one moment that there had been any trauma in her life, at least, nothing serious enough to create a mental block.

As her memories were led down through the years she stopped suddenly at the age of six. I instructed her UNS to bring out the memory which was causing the block and when it did Sheena found herself standing outside a house, too frightened to go inside.

'Whose house is it?' I asked.

'It's my mummy's,' came the hesitant reply.

'Why not go in, then?'

'Because I'm not allowed to make a noise.'

'Why is that, Sheena?'

'Because my daddy has gone away and we are living with my mummy's aunt and uncle. They get very angry if I'm naughty. They keep telling me I mustn't be noisy. Sssh . . .' a finger touched her lips as her voice trailed away.

Amazing though it may appear in hindsight, Sheena's depression all those years later was attributed solely to her mother's request for her not to be noisy. The words preyed on her young mind so much that it blocked off everything that went before. No cruelty whatever had been involved.

That one instruction, repeated time and again during the years the child's elderly relatives lived in the house, had caused a block deep enough to result in depression all these years later. The spasmodic attacks were just the start. Had the block not been removed, Sheena's bouts of depression would have become more frequent and intense, then other symptoms would have followed. Sheena was now able to gain access to all her memories. More pertinently, her bouts of depression ceased and, with the ability to self-heal, she was unlikely to suffer from them ever again.

Those suffering from endogenous depression may not realize it, but the bottled-up memories lodged deep in the mind are not necessarily of major trauma. Incidents which most people would consider trivial can do just as much damage. The death of a pet mouse, being discovered copying homework from a classmate or – like Sheena – being told to be quiet, may not seem very serious but to the child concerned they take on great importance.

These memories are consciously forgotten, but they are stored away at the back of the mind, inhibiting thoughts and actions. If the memory is to function properly and the depression to be lifted, all such barriers must be removed. The sufferer's memories must be directed back in time to uncover each individual event which may be important to present day behaviour.

Patients in a state of deep hypnosis are able to talk of intimate matters which they may not be able to do or may be uncomfortable doing when not under hypnosis, but they do not divulge knowledge they wish to keep to themselves. Private matters remain private.

I always instruct the person whose memory is being restored in this way to remember everything in the waking state, because it is the only way to ensure that the depression and its associated symptoms cause no further trouble. With Sheena, we have seen how a mental barrier formed in childhood resulted from a quite unexpected incident of which she had no conscious memory before being therapeutically regressed.

Sometimes the patient's mind masks the true memory by producing a false one in its place. Leah's block was one such. Her husband Sam described Leah as a moody sort of woman, whose moods bore no relation to anything he could think of, and they were worsening. He had at first attributed them to her age, but now that she was sixty and well past the menopause he began to wonder. The doctor could find no organic cause, and all her physiological tests had proved negative. Here she was, then, at my clinic, confessing that she had an abnormal fear of entering lifts, tunnels, and indeed any confined space.

On the subject of moods there was a difference of opinion between husband and wife. Leah did not see herself as anything but even-tempered. Everybody was entitled to a fit of the blues once in a while, she argued. Sam himself was not as laid-back as he pretended. What she really wanted, she insisted, was help with her fear of confined spaces, which fear she attributed to having spent her childhood in a tiny, cramped apartment, far too small to accommo-date her parents and four siblings with any degree of comfort.

Before putting Leah under hypnosis I questioned her specifically on her phobic history and current problems but nothing else of any significance emerged, just the fear of being confined, she stated. Asked whether any of her brothers and sisters suffered simi-larly she insisted that no, they did not. Regressed to her childhood, Leah suddenly hit a block. She became very agitated and cried pathetically in a manner which suggested she could not have been much more than about three years old.

'No, mummy . . . no . . . the fire. . . .' I waited for a few minutes as she relived the event, then instructed her to return to the present day, leaving behind any pain she may have experienced or illness she may have suffered at the time.

Out of hypnosis Leah now knew the origin of her block and was surprised to find it was not what she had thought. At the age of two-and-a-half the child had been picked up for a cuddle by her mother when, without warning, her mother had suddenly collapsed and dropped her dangerously near the blazing fire. The flames had caught the hem of Leah's dress.

Fortunately her elder brother, who had witnessed the event, had the presence of mind to snatch a rug and wrap it around the terri-fied child, thus smothering the flames before they had a chance to take hold.

Leah had not suffered any pain or injury; it was the act of being virtually smothered in the huge heavy rug that produced her phobia: that, and the fact of her mother's fall. No one in the family had realized that the unfortunate woman had been suffering from an aneurysm. The sudden and unexpected rupturing of a blood vessel was what caused the fatal collapse.

The extent of the horror grew out of all proportion in Leah's mind, but fear of lifts and tunnels turned out to be a 'mask' symp-tom. Although her original explanation was reasonable enough in the circumstances, it was not the real one at all; the root of the problem was so disturbing that she could not even bring her deep-est self to accept it and she offered her own mind a substitute.

The true cause of her trouble was guilt. Leah firmly believed that, because she was in her mother's arms when her mother died, she had been in some way responsible for the death. Now, having relived that day in her far-distant childhood, Leah was told to look at it with mature eyes. Thus she was able to accept the loss of her mother and stop worrying about something over which she had no control.

When she left me her husband drove her to Liverpool, a journey which involved driving through a fairly long tunnel beneath the River Mersey. She reported back to having at first felt a little apprehensive but, trusting her unconscious mind not to let her down and doing a few minutes' self-hypnosis to ensure that she was properly 'psyched-up', she went ahead.

To her great surprise, she felt no fear whatever. Her feelings of guilt and self-recrimination also vanished after that one regression.

I should hate to give the impression that every patient who comes to my door goes away after one session cured of all their physical and mental problems, because that is simply not true, particularly in the cases of those who are suffering from depressive illnesses. The question of whether these patients can be successfully treated or not depends largely on the cause of the depression and how determined they are to rid themselves of it. Some problems can be resolved on the first attempt at regression. For others it involves much mental probing and hard work for both therapist and patient. There are times when the memories are so far out of reach that searching for them is like peeling layers off an onion.

The case of Simon was a very difficult one and very definitely in the 'onion-peeling' category. Simon had been dogged by depression for most of his adult life. He had been on various forms of medication without any success and his sense of hopelessness was so great that he had attempted to kill himself on more than one occasion. His head, he explained, felt as if it consisted of nothing more than a great wodge of cotton wool. He was in a permanent state of confusion.

While Simon admitted that the prescribed medication lifted his depression temporarily, the side-effects produced by the tablets were as bad as the depression itself, sometimes worse. Now he was also having to cope with drowsiness, dry mouth and a general feeling of disorientation. 'The psychiatrist said I was suffering from a serious depressive illness,' he told me, adding that during one period he was completely unable to sleep, while during another he was constantly drowsy.

Certainly, to the uninitiated observer, Simon gave the impression of being slow, lethargic and unwilling to be bothered with anything. It was, of course, the medication which made him like that. 'I can't communicate with people any more. I've lost my job. Now that I'm at home all the time, I know I should be doing odd jobs about the house to help my wife, but I just stand in the kitchen looking at the dishes and the iron and the Hoover. They might as well be Everest as far as I'm concerned. It's hopeless. I keep telling myself this is stupid, and I should pull myself up by the bootstraps, but I can't. Believe me, I can't.'

I did believe him; I *knew* he could not. But I told him that even with the proverbial boots still on he had taken a very positive step in coming to see me. Where did he think his problems had begun, I asked: had he any conscious memory of an event, or events, which might have caused his depression?

He thought long and hard before coming up with the suggestion that it might be related to his schooldays. Every term when exams were imminent his brain seized up. He went on to explain that he was one of the youngest boys in the class, intellectually bright, but physically immature. A puny sort of child, Simon had difficulty in making friends and became a prime target for bullying. Despite his flair for music, art and languages, he had one blind spot: mathematics. He was not keen on traditional male sports either, as a result of which his peers regarded him as something of a sissy. 'I managed to gain a university place to study arts and philosophy, but "totally flipped", and never took it up.

'Instead, I found an office job which bored me to tears and I ended up even more unhappy than I had been at school. The doctor sent me to a psychotherapist; I had three years' counselling and at the end of it all the conclusion that we came to was that I'd been bullied, which was something I already knew. I was sent on a course in anxiety management, then another on assertiveness training. None of it was any good. That was when they started bombarding me with tablets and the dosage was increased with every visit.' Somehow, he still managed to get by and to pursue some of his hobbies and interests. 'I met my wife, Debbie, at our local chamber music society. She's very supportive but the marriage isn't working because I find the responsibility overwhelming. I do love Debbie, but I'm afraid she'll leave me. I'm so unhappy.'

Simon entered hypnosis more easily than I had anticipated. He regressed to senior school without too much difficulty but hit a problem in the juniors.

'Can't do sums,' came the whimpered remark. 'Teacher's putting big black crosses on my book and everyone's laughing 'cos nobody else has big black crosses.'

'Is the teacher not showing you how to do your sums?' I ventured.

'No.'

'What's on the blackboard, then?'

'More sums . . . don't understand them.'

'Then ask the teacher to explain them to you.'

'Can't,' came the distressed reply. 'She's shouting at me . . . stupid boy . . . stupid boy . . . she's horrible . . . she's going to get me.'

'How is she going to get you?'

'After school. Have to stay in after school when the others have gone home. She's shouting at me again. . . I don't know . . . don't. . . .' The experience was proving very distressing, but there were still no tears. 'No, miss . . . no . . .'

'Simon, I want you to remember . . .' I instructed the man under hypnosis. 'Remember. It's only when you remember all the emotions that you'll get rid of this problem. So, come on, remember. I can't help you if you don't go through it properly.'

I made strenuous efforts to try and determine what exactly was at the root of his problem, but the only response was his repeated words. 'Stupid boy. . .'

I tried another method.

'It's not you who's stupid. It's the teacher. Teachers are supposed to explain things to their pupils. If she doesn't show you how to do your sums, how can you do them? What's wrong with asking for help? Everyone needs help.'

At long last tears began to appear on the face of the patient.

'You won't be smacked for crying . . . let them flow,' I urged. 'Tears are a release. It is not weak to cry.'

'Little boys don't cry . . . stupid, lazy baby, she says. The other boys keep calling me a sissy.'

'Simon,' I insist. 'You are *not* a sissy. Little boys do cry . . . should cry . . . so come on, let the tears flow.'

'But I'm frightened of the teacher,' he blurted out. And there it was, at last. He was frightened of his maths teacher. It took five long sessions before we finally hit the real cause of his problem.

Simon did come back some weeks later, this time accompanied by Debbie, who told me quietly that she had never had any intention of leaving him. With that worry out of the way I wanted to satisfy myself that Simon's problem really was resolved and that he was practising self-hypnosis properly in order to heal his mind of the hurt which that appalling teacher had caused. I was pleased to find everything in order.

As an exercise I threw out a question to all those present in the room. 'What,' I asked 'does happiness mean to you?'

The answers were as varied as those who provided them.

'Being fulfilled,' said one man. 'Having food in my stomach and cash in my pocket,' said another. 'Success,' said a third. 'Being able to enjoy good food and wine. . . . Walking my dog in the country-side. . . . Listening to Beethoven. . . .' the answers came thick and fast. When I reached Simon, he paused a few minutes, then smiled broadly and I realized it was the first time I had seen him do so.

His answer was both enlightening and rewarding.

'Happiness,' he told the assembled company 'is never having to take antidepressants again.'

Simon explained to the others how the practice of self-hypnosis was helping him. To me, he mentioned that his timing was not very good. 'When I put myself into hypnosis for ten minutes, I sometimes overrun to twelve or fifteen. Once, it was almost twenty.'

That, I told him, was because he had had considerable stress building up over the years.

'You must trust your own mind,' I added. 'After a while, when your body grows accustomed to relaxing, it will level itself out. Don't worry about it. You're doing very well.

'Eventually, you'll be accurate to within a fraction of a second.'

Long-term hurt

Minds which have been hurt persistently over a long period of time take much longer to heal. Years, decades, of suffering from low self-esteem cannot be eradicated overnight. Sue Harper's case was one such.

In some respects, Sue's story is similar to Simon's; in others, it is very different. It is similar in that she too has been blighted by depression and in almost total withdrawal from most forms of human contact. She too had bad experiences in childhood. Her case is different from Simon's in that her depression had an added factor: eating problems.

Sue, who is in her early forties, unmarried and living with friends in Wales, is a very articulate person and was anxious to relate her own story. 'I always thought my trouble started with anorexia,' she told me. 'The anorexia led to bulimia and, as my depression worsened, so did my reaction to it.

'I developed behavioural problems: inflicting injury on myself, cutting my arms until they were just a mass of lacerations. I was in and out of hospital so often I've lost count. Long-term psychiatric care involved heavy sedation. At one stage, I was on thirty-two tablets a day; and during another short period of time I had a total of thirteen doses of electro-convulsive therapy. I began to feel a zombie.

'The pathetic thing about it was that I hadn't a clue what was causing the depression. I thought I was born that way: a freak of nature. I never realized I was suffering from any form of illness.

'After all, I looked perfectly healthy and as far as other people were concerned there was nothing wrong with me. At home and at school my low opinion of myself was reinforced. One of the nuns who taught me called me a lazy fat lump; an accusation which, to the sensitive child I was, shattered my confidence and nearly broke my heart.'

Add the concept of the unpleasant and thoroughly insensitive teacher to the accusation of being lazy, and what do you get? No, it does not take three guesses; the scenario is all too familiar.

Yet the major cause of Sue's depression was something entirely different and came to light quite by accident. As occasionally happens, this patient was one of a group waiting to try hypnosis when something strange happened. Another patient was being treated, but it was Sue who began to cry.

'Suddenly, and quite spontaneously, several old memories flooded my mind: incidents and experiences that had been locked away inside me for years,' she reflected later.

'When I was under hypnosis for my own treatment you told me I didn't have to reveal any private thoughts, but I must remember them, accept them for what they were, and discard them. The future was what mattered, you insisted, not the past.

'I had a good cry, but didn't want to talk to anyone about what I had been through. I've thought about it a lot but, if you don't mind, it's such a deeply personal matter that I would rather not disclose the details here, either.

'I'd prefer to focus on the positive aspects and say that since learning self-hypnosis, I've stopped injuring myself and feel much better. I really do believe you helped me then, and continue to help me now: both mentally and physically.'

Because Sue's depression had been so deep, so persistent, she needed several sessions of hypnotherapy before she was able to cope with self-hypnosis. Even then I felt it necessary to give Sister Poacher the ability to induce Sue into hypnosis for those occasions when she could not manage on her own.

As with other patients who have been helped in this way, the transference is proving eminently suitable for Sue.

'If I'm really stressed-out and so low that I can't get into the right state of mind to help myself, Gwyneth helps me the way you taught her to,' she reflected. 'Naturally, I still have days when I feel down. With me, I suppose it's control at the moment, because the actual cure will take time.'

Sue has been practising self-hypnosis relatively successfully now since 1993; she tells me she also finds aromatherapy relaxing.

'But if it hadn't been for the fact that both Gwyneth and yourself felt there was something worth fighting for, I wouldn't be here today. Self-hypnosis has given me the stability missing from my life for so long. At last I can stop regarding myself as a freak because I know now that I'm just an ordinary, average human being, like everyone else. More importantly, I know I am loved and wanted. My ultimate aim is to contribute something worthwhile to society, so that one day I might be able to help others in a similar situation.'

11 Guilt

At least several billion years have passed since the first simple life forms were created. Early vertebrate embryos had skin, muscles and blood. As the long process of evolution by natural selection continued from one generation to the next, we developed an increasingly profound and positive view of life. We also developed the ability to cope with it.

One would think that, after all this time, we would be well attuned to our mental processes, yet nothing could be further from the truth. Our patterns of behaviour have strayed so far from those of our primitive forebears that in terms of mental development we could, speaking evolutionarily, be back in the Dark Ages.

Retrieving data from our memory banks

Convoluted maze though our mind undoubtedly is, it is not impenetrable. Much earlier in this book reference was made to the incalculable amount of data accumulated and stored by our mental computer, all of which data should be accessible at any given time. Because our unconscious mind is the one link we retain with our ancient ancestors, it alone can relate to the built-in mechanisms by which cells developed to make us what we are. The blueprint is there for us to extract what we will. All we have to do is tap into it.

The internal computer controls our daily living according to instructions which have been and are continuing to be fed into it. But the information disk containing the program can sometimes slip out of step. When it does it must be readjusted.

One of the great mysteries of our mind is its amazing ability to allow errors in the code to be rectified, so that we can be put back on track. My function as a therapist is not to unravel the mysteries of the human mind, but to teach patients how to adjust the function of their thinking, in order to unravel their *own* mental entanglements.

Abortion

Take abortion, for example, a subject which is contentious, controversial and *very* emotive. On the one hand we have the pro-life moralists and theologians, on the other the pro-choice reformers and women's groups. It is not my intention to discuss the merits or demerits of either viewpoint because in my considered opinion the issue goes deeper than most people could ever imagine. It stretches right back to those biological processes which have made women what they are. It relates to an entire system which is geared towards the preservation of life, not its destruction; a gut instinct, I suppose it could be called. After all, the prime motivation in *every* form of life is reproduction and continuation of the species.

For millennia, females of most species have produced and protected their young: an instinct so deeply rooted that it has become part of our birthright. The whole concept of woman's design is to propagate the species, to carry young and to give birth.

One cannot expect a natural instinct to be eradicated immediately by a modern, man-made law. So, when it comes to the matter of foetal development, some sort of unconscious reaction is inevitable. Abortion, being fraught with so many ethical dilemmas, can have a major impact on the mind of the individual concerned. Therapists called upon to treat guilt and other deep-rooted reactions must understand and be sensitive to whatever psychological needs such patients might present.

Individual cases (Eleanor, Angela, Jennie)

To illustrate the point, allow me to introduce three young women. I shall call them Eleanor, Angela and Jennie. Those are not their real names, but everything else about them is genuine and the reports

I am about to present are accurate representations of their case histories.

Eleanor was twenty-nine years old, recently married, and her approach was by way of an enquiry. Could hypnosis help solve her marital difficulties, she wondered. I invited this young woman, as I invite all potential patients, to bring along a relative or friend to make her feel more relaxed about the idea of undergoing hypnotherapy, but she declined. No one else knew about her problem, she averred, and she would prefer to keep it that way. On arrival at the clinic Eleanor explained that the reason for her reticence was because she was unable to achieve an orgasm. This upset her far more deeply than such a relatively common condition might seem to warrant, particularly in someone who had only been married for a few months.

In regression all went well until an attempt at sending her back through her memories spotlighted the underlying cause of her trouble. Suddenly, she became distraught and cried out, 'I've murdered my baby.' I let her continue weeping until I felt she had accepted the memories she had previously repressed. The abortion had been carried out some years earlier and while one part of her mind had rejected the event the other part was reacting to it.

Eleanor's abortion had been recommended by her doctor and had been quite legal. She had agreed with the decision (she thought) but under hypnosis she showed that she had not. Her present difficulties had come about because of that ancient primeval instinct. In other words, the unconscious part of her mind had registered its objection in the strongest possible way. Asked if she now practised birth control, Eleanor assured me that she did. When asked whether she considered termination of pregnancy to be merely carrying the practice a stage further, her answer was again in the affirmative.

This enabled her to view her present predicament rather differently. Eleanor returned to my clinic some weeks later to say that she and her husband were now enjoying a full and satisfactory sex life and there had been no further problems. Eleanor's case was the easiest of the three to resolve because she did not have any strong religious convictions to get in the way, whereas Angela and Jennie were both of Irish Catholic extraction and steeped in the tenets of their Church.

Angela's husband must have been one of the most patient men around. Despite the fact that the couple had been together for six months and were very much in love, the marriage had still not been consummated. Angela's privately professed difficulty was that she could not bear her husband to touch her in bed. She further explained that the unfortunate man assumed she was still a virgin and that time would resolve her problem. Angela did not disillusion him and the whole scenario was causing a psychological tug of war in her mind. By the time she came to me her emotions were in crisis.

Under deep hypnosis, Angela regressed easily to the age of fifteen, when her memories came to an abrupt halt. The mental turmoil she had been experiencing originated in some rather crude attempts to abort a baby she had been carrying. The then teenager's methods involved a steel knitting needle and a bucket. Her botched abortion caused a haemorrhage so severe that it endangered her life. She was fortunate in that the self-inflicted damage did not render her infertile; it did, however, make her incapable of ever being able to give birth by natural means.

Angela's interpretation of the mental anguish she experienced as a result was that God was punishing her. In passing, she mentioned that she had, of course, confessed and been absolved of her sin, so that as far as her faith was concerned, eternal damnation was no longer a threat. She was at a loss to know why her misdeed was still affecting her, why she was still in torment.

Keeping the problem in the religious context in which the patient had firmly placed it, I thought it might be appropriate to suggest that God, having 'cleansed' her soul, might want her to go ahead and do the same with her mind. If He had forgiven her, did she not think the time was right for her to forgive herself? I also reminded her that the exclusion of her disturbing unconscious memory from her conscious mind was jeopardizing her health. Put like that, she said, she had to agree. She could appreciate that painful though bringing the memory into the forefront of her mind had proved, she already felt better, but as far as I was concerned she was still much too reserved about the whole experience.

Her lack of tears showed she was still blotting out a vital aspect of it. Regressed once more to her moment of trauma, she relived the event, this time with all its accompanying emotions. When at last she burst into tears I knew she was there. This time she really did bring out all the painful memories. Now at last her mind was clear. She should have no further trouble.

I did not expect to hear from Angela again. But a year or so later I received a greetings card announcing the arrival (by caesarian section) of a healthy baby son. I do not know if she ever told her husband what was at the root of her earlier problem. Whatever I might have thought about the deception, I kept my opinion to myself because it is not my place to be judgemental. As far as I was concerned, the entire episode was over and done with; Angela's mental block had been cleared. Her private life was no longer any of my business.

Jennie was in her thirties, married with several small children, a husband declared redundant from his former job, a mortgage and rapidly mounting debts. When it all became too much, she sank into a state of deep depression and was actually referred to me by her GP. Not wishing to prescribe long-term medication, he thought hypnotherapy worth trying. Outlining the background to her case, the doctor explained that Jennie had had some gynaecological problems. He further explained that his patient had no objection to my knowing that, on medical grounds, one of her pregnancies had been legally terminated and sterilization suggested to avoid further problems. But the patient had said no with the result that six months later she was pregnant again. Only this time she lost the foetus through natural causes.

Jennie remembered all of this before regression, which made me wonder if her depression might relate to something else. But no. We were back with the same old problem, as I discovered when she regressed.

It is significant that the cry coming from the depths of her UNS was exactly the same as that of Angela: each mother accusing herself of 'murdering' her unborn baby, each weighed down by the burden of her guilt. Because Jennie's background and upbringing were so similar to those of Angela, she benefited from a similar course of therapy and her problems have also been resolved. These three cases demonstrate how the ancient voice of our forebears still resounds in each of us. It enables us to pinpoint and remove problems deep in the mind, even those attacking the very core of our being.

Failing as mothers? (Suzanne, Mrs T., Mrs L.)

Suzanne's reason for requesting therapy was because she claimed she was failing as a mother. At first when this middle-aged woman began to regress, I thought that what we were faced with might be more of the same, but it was not quite that. Suzanne thought she had completed her family until she found herself pregnant for the fifth time. Her first reaction was indeed to abort the foetus, and with that in mind she drank rather too much gin and kept soaking herself in very hot baths, to no avail. Even the strenuous effort of moving various heavy appliances around her kitchen failed to achieve the required effect. As the regression continued details of her history emerged. Suzanne went full-term without difficulty to produce a fine, healthy daughter but the sheer beauty of her newborn infant brought on a great big dose of guilt.

The new mother kept asking herself how she could possibly have considered disposing of her precious daughter in such a cavalier fashion. Unable to reconcile herself with the power of her own emotional feelings, Suzanne lavished attention on her youngest child and completely spoilt her. As the little girl grew up, her mother tried to redress the balance by favouring the child over her four older siblings. But nothing would assuage Suzanne's guilt: the mental flagellation went on and on. While this woman's prime source of guilt was directly related to her erstwhile attempts to 'kill' her baby, it branched out in another way. Now she was also accusing herself of being 'a rotten mother'. It was up to me to make her see reason. Today, with most of her family grown up, how were they all faring, I asked.

'The eldest son's a builder, my daughter's a legal secretary, the next son's at university doing media studies and the youngest two are still at school,' she told me.

'And the daughter you've been feeling so guilty about?' I asked.

A broad smile lit up the face of this full-time mother-of-five: 'She's twelve next week. A lovely girl, and very sporty. She has lots of medals for swimming. Look. . . .' From her bag, the mother produced a photograph of a pretty little girl in a swim suit.

'You must be very proud of her achievements.'

'I am. I'm proud of them all,' she announced.

'Right then, you've done your best for your family,' I told her. 'Can't you see that your children wouldn't have managed so well without your constant support and encouragement?'

She paused briefly before responding: 'I suppose.'

'So why on earth should you consider yourself a failure?' I insisted.

Looked at in that light, Suzanne grudgingly acknowledged that perhaps she was not such a bad mother after all. I gave her therapy to restore her confidence and taught her how to remove any feelings of self-doubt if they should ever threaten in future. She went away happy.

Two other mothers who saw themselves as failures were Mrs T., a young career woman and mother of twins and Mrs L., an elderly widow with one daughter. Before going under hypnosis Mrs T. felt it necessary to tell me something of her habits.

When the children were babies it had been her custom to leave them with a child-minder as early as possible every morning and she deeply regretted the fact that circumstances prevented her ever being able to collect them until just before their bedtime. She felt that by pursuing her accountancy studies she had more or less abdicated her maternal duties. The twins were now at school and, because she was holding down a high-powered executive position, she was still juggling with work and home to provide responsibly for her children, which meant she still saw considerably less of them than she would have wished.

Mrs. L's case was rather different. Having been blasted by the media with alarming news stories about recent findings in relation to childhood cruelty and having heard all the arguments in favour of today's softly-softly approach, she had found herself wondering if the slaps given to chastize her own daughter might spoil that daughter's chance of happy parenthood.

Despite the dissimilarity of these two cases, I used a similar approach for Mrs T. and Mrs L., questioning them about their respective children in the way that I had questioned Suzanne about the young daughter whose birth had been surrounded by such guilt. In so doing I learned that the twins were doing remarkably well at school and had actually won several class and sporting prizes. Mrs L's daughter was a well-adjusted young woman now pursuing her own career, never having been a disruptive child, dabbled in drugs, or caused her mother any concern whatsoever. There was no reason to suppose the younger woman would be any less successful as a wife or mother.

We all worry about the people we love and parents find it particularly difficult to take anything other than a subjective view of their children. Sometimes it needs an outsider to put matters in their proper perspective. Despite the fact that these two mothers found it difficult to come to terms with their respective situations, they were each coping admirably.

Inability to grieve

Guilt is not an exclusively female phenomenon. One case of guilt I encountered in a man was that of Brian P. Brian had lost his wife almost a year before his visit to me.

He came because he was suffering from depression and an inability to grieve. I offered my condolences and told him I would do what I could. Brian went on to explain that what upset him most was not just the inability to grieve but the lack of memories about the death itself. Although he had a vague feeling that his wife had died tragically, he was unable to recall the full circumstances surrounding the event.

For some unknown reason Brian blamed himself for his wife's demise. Could I help him overcome his feelings, he asked? I could try, I told him; though I did wonder what possible motivation this man could have for believing himself responsible. Brian's brain was refusing to allow him to remember the events surrounding his wife's death. The shock had triggered something in his mind which repressed his unconscious memories, totally excluding them from his conscious. It was as if the door connecting conscious and unconscious memories had somehow been snapped shut. With no control over the situation, he had called upon my help.

Because Brian was under such great stress, I did think he might have had some difficulty in entering hypnosis, but he had none at all and regression to the event showed that he had been blaming himself, quite wrongly. Here are the facts as they emerged from the depths of this patient's unconscious mind. Mrs P. had been innocently cycling home from the shops when a car swerved directly into her path; the force of the impact caused a crushed skull, severe internal injuries and multiple lacerations throughout her body.

Still under deep hypnosis, Brian relived the events, recounting how his wife had been rushed to hospital deeply unconscious, in which state she remained for several months. Tubes were the only things keeping her alive. She was in what doctors describe as a permanent vegetative state. In other words she was suffering a living death, yet Brian spent long, tearful hours at his inert wife's bedside, holding her hands, telling her over and again that he loved her and always would.

When it was finally agreed by an independent team of doctors that there would never be any improvement in the patient's condition, the consultant in charge of her case suggested to Brian that artificial feeding should be withdrawn to enable his wife to end her life peacefully and with dignity. The comatose patient would be made comfortable but she would be given nothing to either prevent or accelerate her death because she was, in effect, already dead. All the medical guidelines were met, and after considerable praying and heart-searching, Brian eventually agreed to the consultant's suggestion. It was then that guilt set in, swiftly followed by depression, both of which hit him particularly badly after the funeral.

The effect on his system was cumulative. He could not grieve properly because of his guilt; the guilt caused insomnia and loss of appetite. He became lethargic and depressed. The doctor prescribed antidepressants, which apparently helped on a temporary basis; at least, they enabled Brian to keep his emotions so well under cover that no one suspected what he was going through. With the assistance of his medication Brian coped, working long hours, pushing himself to his limits in the office because there was nothing to go home to.

Indeed, he managed so well that his boss offered him promotion. That brought on a whole new kind of guilt, because it had never happened in his wife's lifetime and was the type of promotion which would have made her proud and happy. Still under hypnosis and deep in regression, Brian was able to view the situation in its true light and to see that he was in no way responsible for his wife's death. There was nothing more he could have done.

I felt it necessary to instil a positive message in his mind: 'You are young,' I told him. 'You are strong. You must keep yourself healthy and never feel guilty again. Your wife loved you and she knew that you loved her. She would not want you to make yourself ill in this way.' Freed from his anxieties, he agreed that he had renewed purpose to his life.

Dealing with Brian's problems by means of regression helped him rid himself of all those potent negative emotions and enabled him to begin the grieving process. With his memory pathway clear, he would be able to remember his wife in a more positive, loving way, and to appreciate that he had done everything within his power to help her.

The daily practice of self-hypnosis would enable him to keep on top of the situation and to think in more positive terms.

The student nurse

Recalling Brian's problem and how it was resolved brings another hospital-related case to mind. This one concerns a very successful nursing sister who came to me with a curious problem.

The woman, whom I shall call Sister X said that although she was acknowledged as a highly skilled person who ran her professional life with ease and efficiency, her private life was rather different. What concerned Sister X was that she could not put her finger on precisely what was wrong.

'I'm sorry,' she said, 'but that's how it is. I spend half my life apologizing, but have no idea what I'm apologizing for. Does that make sense to you?'

It did not, I told her, but it might if she were to regress to whatever sparked off this unconscious guilt. Before undergoing regression, was she *sure* there was nothing she could recall consciously which might be associated with it? Not a thing, she insisted. So, having induced her into hypnosis and led her memories back in the usual manner, we went right down her nursing years to the days before she was a sister, to being a staff nurse, a nurse in a general ward, then into her student days and *wham* . . . there it was. A big black nothing. No earlier memories.

That mental block took some getting through. What transpired when we eventually managed to see daylight was that the then Student Nurse X had been left to do a routine check on a seriously ill young patient in the ward where she was helping out. When she drew back the curtains surrounding his bed, she recognized the signs of respiratory failure and was alert enough to know that the boy was dangerously ill. Not knowing quite how to cope with a situation which was totally alien to her, she raced from the bedside to fetch a doctor. But by the time she returned, which could not have been more than a minute or two later, the patient was dead.

The student nurse blamed herself absolutely for the death of her young patient and never forgave herself for not taking more positive action at the time. Because it had been such a dreadful experience her unconscious mind had erased the memory from her conscious, which was why she had such negative repercussions. Still under hypnosis, but now aware of why she had spent her intervening years virtually apologizing for living, Sister X needed one basic fact to be pointed out.

'You were only a student,' I reminded her. 'How could you be expected to handle such a serious situation? If there is any blame to be attached here it should be placed firmly at the door of whoever left you alone in that ward, when you had neither the training nor the experience to cope with a dying patient.'

Yes, she acknowledged the fact, now. Furthermore, in her present role, she would ensure that no student nurse in her care would ever be faced with such a crisis. Thus was another block successfully removed.

Forgetting to pay

Guilt is not necessarily associated with major trauma. With this, as with other sentiments and emotions, silly little incidents can cause the mind to block off its memories. One woman's guilt was found to have originated after a shopping expedition, when she recalled standing outside a shop, looking at the contents of her bag in horror. It contained a tin of corned beef for which she had not paid. In regression, she kept repeating the words: 'I stole . . . I stole . . . I stole. . . .'

Believe me, that woman took some convincing that this was *not* theft, merely an oversight. It was certainly not just cause for making herself ill. We got there in the end and this patient had no further recurrence of her guilt.

There we are, then. In media circles, because I am known chiefly for my work in the field of age-regressions, I am invariably described as a 'pre-life regressionist' or sometimes, more colourfully, as the 'time tunnel man'; but pre-birth blocks account for only a very small proportion of the mental blocks I am called upon to remove.

Most originate in the patient's own lifetime, particularly those causing fears and phobias. When it comes to targeting the root of those fears and phobias, regression is a powerful therapeutic weapon and it yields *results* as we shall see in the next chapter.

12   Fears and Phobias

Difference between the two

Question: What is the difference between a fear and a phobia?

Answer: Fear is a straightforward emotion which everyone experiences when confronted with a threat of some kind: redundancy, illness, death. A phobia is an illogical terror of something commonplace like an innocent kitten, a motor car, or a daily newspaper. A fear is logical, a phobia is quite illogical and is invariably due to some long-standing experience, or experiences, which cannot be recalled consciously.

Put like that, it sounds cold and clinical but, believe me, the phobic patient can go through absolute hell. The difficulty is that other people (some doctors included) tend to dismiss these enigmatic fears through sheer lack of understanding. People who are blind, have fractured limbs, or visible wounds of one type or another are in a different category. Their problems can be *seen* and therefore understood. Those suffering from phobias must go through their agony alone. Mentioning an irrational fear to a non-phobic person often results in dismissal or derision. Family, friends and colleagues are likely to turn the matter into a subject of fun. Doctors – unless they have experienced some sort of phobia themselves – are confused because phobic patients have such difficulty putting their views across. In the absence of visible or palpable signs, the average general practitioner is unsure what he is up against.

How often, I wonder, have the words 'It's all in the mind' been uttered on such occasions? *Of course* a phobia is all in the mind; where it is *not* is in the imagination, which is the implied criticism.

What people may not realize is how insidious the effects of that phobia can be on our entire system. It is not unusual for doctors to prescribe antidepressants or tranquillizers for such patients but they know full well that these medications simply suppress the system. Some doctors would argue that antidepressants and tranquillizers are prescribed in order to prevent overreation in their patients, but the distressing side-effects of such medications can prove as bad as, if not worse than, the phobia itself. Who wants to risk constipation, a dry mouth, urine retention, blurred vision, palpitations, on *top* of a phobia?

Admittedly, the average medical professional does acknowledge the existence of a phobia but, more often than not, has no concept of its inherent danger to general health. The phobic sufferer, therefore, tired of being met with negative attitudes, tends to give up discussing the subject. The sight of disbelief, even amusement, registering on people's faces is just too hurtful. Are they really as stupid and inadequate as people seem to be suggesting? Is their mind playing tricks on them?

All too often the outcome is that they stop asking for help. That is a great pity because patients who respond to hypnosis will find that regressive therapy can get right down to the root of the problem, to dispose of it once and for all.

Lifts (elevators)

Penny Y. and Roz H. visited me together. Colleagues and friends, despite their age difference (Penny was twenty-three years old, Roz forty-eight), they had come because of Roz's depression. Associated with the depression was a pathological fear of lifts. Penny could sympathize with her friend because she was equally terrified of rope bridges, but without the associated depression. Having been obliged to walk along one across a ravine during a childhood holiday with her parents, she remembered the incident all too clearly and now, despite living near just such a bridge in Chester, avoided the things like the plague. Bridges in general did not bother her, she added. That is a straightforward fear and a rational response to it. Penny had no need of therapy.

Roz's fear, on the other hand, was completely irrational. Unlike Penny, she had no conscious memory of any incident which might have triggered it off. Nothing would persuade her to enter a lift, or anything similar, yet the very thought of having to do so sent shivers down her spine. That is a phobia.

Phobias can be straightforward, or they can be extremely complex. Straightforward phobias are caused by one traumatic episode in the patient's life and when that is attended to – usually during a single session of regressive hypnotherapy – the phobia is no more. The complex variety are much more difficult and time-consuming. Removal of multiple phobias takes many sessions, conducted over a period of weeks or months even, depending on the circumstances.

Roz H.'s phobia was not unusual; its cause and treatment will be examined presently. Curiously enough, fear of lifts, or elevators, is one which does crop up from time to time and we saw (chapter 10) what had caused Leah's phobia and how they had affected it until regressive hypnotherapy made her confront her trauma and dispose of it.

Motor cars

An irrational fear of travelling in motor cars (and, for that matter, buses and trains), while not exactly commonplace, is another one which manifests itself from time to time. There are various reasons why people fear car travel and we met some of these sufferers (also in chapter 10).

Janet M., an otherwise sensible housewife, refused point blank to step inside a motor car of any type, private or commercial. She did not possess a car and positively refused to ride in those of her friends. Even taxis were taboo. It was all very inconvenient but she got by, alternating between walking, riding her bicycle and using public transport. As is so often the case with such phobias, Janet also suffered from claustrophobia and presumed she was stuck with her two problems for the rest of her days. Then she heard of a neighbour whose spider phobia had been successfully treated by hypnosis and wondered if her phobia would also respond to treatment.

As a matter of fact, it did: and what a fascinating case it turned out to be. Janet, who looked nothing like her admitted age of fifty-nine, regressed to wartime Britain, when she was living in a Bristol suburb. Her mental block originated during a car journey from her home city to visit friends in Cardiff.

The vehicle had just entered the Severn Tunnel when it was, to quote Janet herself 'as if all hell broke loose'. Enemy aircraft could be heard overhead, bombs rained down, the sudden explosion making everything in the tunnel vibrate. Janet, who was a small child at the time, did not understand what was happening and was terrified. To make matters worse, her parents' vehicle and all those others already in the tunnel were trapped inside for several hours. Janet's block was duly removed and, yes, she is now perfectly well able to travel in any type of vehicle.

Performing in public

Earlier in the book I referred to the many students at schools, colleges of education and universities who come to the clinic in order to be helped with their examinations. Ego-boosting therapy is called for in a variety of situations.

The problem for one gifted music student related to a specific situation. The student, who asked me to refer to her only as Estelle (it is not her real name), hopes to become a concert pianist and, although happy for her problem to be reported, does not wish it to come back and haunt her when she reaches the peak of her career, as she undoubtedly will before long. Her chosen pseudonym is significant: it means 'star'.

Estelle told me that the general consensus of opinion was that she played very well in concerts and recitals organized by her college. That, she explained, was because she knew everyone in the audience, so felt reasonably confident. She even appeared, on one memorable occasion, as guest soloist with a large symphony orchestra based in the same city as her music academy. That did not shake her confidence either.

The stage was lit but the auditorium was in darkness; therefore, not being able to see the rows of concert-goers facing her, she played as she would to a group of friends. Despite her undoubted talent, Estelle was terrified at the idea of facing large numbers of people and, as a result, worried about future instrumental performances. The thought of playing to strangers in a situation where she could see them made her freeze: in a church hall, for example, or at an open-air concert. It created a false situation in her mind: she felt her inexperience would be apparent to all those music-lovers and that she would see disappointment register on the mass of faces confronting her.

Estelle worried, too, that her lack of confidence might spill over to the keyboard and make her strike wrong notes. If that happened, she vowed she would give up the idea of a concert career, even though she loved playing so much and such a career would be the fulfillment of her life's ambitions. She had no wish to be a second- or third-rate performer; she would give up all her hopes and dreams if she could not reach the peak of her profession. Estelle's sole ambition was to live up to her adopted name: she wanted to be a star.

'But last week was a nightmare.'

She told me about a charity performance she had given in a church, with all lights blazing. 'I could see hundreds of people sitting there waiting for me to start, wanting their money's worth and my nerves were shot to pieces. I made such a hash of that recital that now I'm terrified someone will tell the college principal how awful I was and demand their money back. Then I shall be sent down.'

Poor Estelle. She *was* in a state.

'Did the audience in the church applaud your performance?'

'Yes, but they would anyway, as a matter of courtesy.'

'Were there any disparaging remarks at the time?'

'No. Everyone was very sweet. They wanted an encore, and presented me with a big bouquet of flowers afterwards.'

'Hmmm . . .' I mused. 'They'd hardly have responded so positively if you had, as you say, made such a hash of your playing.'

'You weren't there,' she responded, still not convinced.

Having listened sympathetically to everything Estelle said, I concluded that her fear was feeding on itself and was in danger of becoming a self-fulfilling prophecy. What she needed more than anything else was to have her confidence boosted. Estelle, a bright girl, responded almost instantaneously to the hypnotic induction and quickly learned the technique of self-treatment. As I do with all my patients, I advised her to practise every day and gave her a set of my specially printed cards. She was to instruct her own unconscious mind to restore her self-confidence and never allow it to slip again.

By telling herself: 'I am now going to relax for ten minutes and when I come back, I will feel fully confident to play my best, whatever the circumstances or conditions,' her panic attacks would vanish. Before giving any performance, she should again put herself into a state of self-hypnosis for at least ten minutes and use the same words. The more we nag our UNS, the more likely it is to get the message. While Estelle was in her state of deep relaxation I told her to repeat the following words after me: 'You, my unconscious mind, will not allow me to have any more fear of performing in public.

'It doesn't matter whether the lights are on or off, whether I am playing to a large number of people, or just a few, I must always play to the best of my ability.'

I suggested that she give her UNS this instruction before every performance, to ensure its success. Then I told her: 'You are young, attractive and a gifted musician. You are perfectly capable of performing in public or tackling any other aspect of your work. Initial nervousness is natural, but you will grow more confident daily. In this way you will gain the respect and admiration of all your audiences, whatever the setting. You will relax and enjoy everything to do with your work. You are a talented pianist. Your college principal knows it. You know it. I know it. You must see that your audience knows it too.'

After that single hypnotic session, Estelle began to play with confidence. Her fears subsided and the concept of *seeing* those who had come to her performances switched from being a frightening experience to an eminently pleasurable one. Today, she is well on her way to the stardom she craves.

Making decisions

Fear of making decisions or, having made them, those decisions being wrong, can cause untold disturbance in the mind, particularly when associated with long-term insecurity. This fear was what brought Miss O'G. to my clinic. She had just been promoted to an important managerial post as an accounts executive. Her problem was that when under stress she pulled out great chunks of her hair. The more stressed she became, the more hair she removed.

In regression, Miss O'G.'s problem was found to have originated some years earlier. She had left school without any academic qualifications and, despite (or perhaps *because* of) the deficit, had made a remarkable success of her life. She had scaled the career ladder by means of sheer hard work and determination.

A first-class saleswoman, she had been promoted rapidly until here she was, on the brink of being made a company director, earning a much higher salary than would have been possible had she passed her examinations and taken up some academic career. Learning self-hypnosis to boost her confidence put this patient right back on track. Today, Miss O'G. is relaxed, she has stopped pulling her hair out and is holding down her new post with flair and skill, fully equipped to make any major decisions her highly-paid position might demand. Last time I heard from her she was working in the City of London, making vast amounts of money buying and selling commodities, which is hardly the type of career she could pursue if frightened of making decisions.

Flying

Mr McK. and Miss J. consulted me because of their fear of flying. These two visited me on separate occasions and did not know each other. I present them together merely as a couple of individual case histories extracted from my files.

For Mr McK. his problem had an added nuisance factor, because this man *needed* to fly on a fairly regular basis. He worked as marketing manager, promoting software for an international company of computer manufacturers.

He could not recall any specific incident which might have sparked off his fear. None of his colleagues were aware of his problem; he hid it well, he was ashamed of it. But he was also intelligent enough to know that somewhere deep in the storage vaults of his memory banks there must be a causative factor. Regression proved his assumption to be correct.

Mr Mck.'s memories were clear for some years until we hit a block at the age of nineteen, when it was as if the words 'access restricted' had come up on his mental screen. After the usual form of treatment, this man's repressed memory turned out to be related to an incident on board a holiday jet bound for the Far East, which involved a brief stopover at Amsterdam. As the aircraft prepared for landing there was an unexpected change in air pressure, with the result that Mr McK. experienced a blinding headache, a sensation of suffocation and the firm belief that by the time the plane touched down at Schiphol – if it ever did – he would be dead.

Similarly, Miss J.'s fear of flying related to a specific incident when she was a passenger on board a holiday flight. Her block was formed *en route* from Liverpool to the Isle of Man when 'for technical reasons', the aircraft had to return to Speke. The situation took on a more sinister aspect when the stewardess began preparing passengers for a belly landing on foam. As the aircraft began its descent and the runway came into view fire engines could be seen standing by. The runway had been cleared and it was obvious to everyone on board that the airport was on full alert.

It was subsequently revealed that the instrument panel had shown the plane to be coming in with faulty landing gear, although the 'emergency' turned out to be nothing more serious than an electrical fault, which had produced an incorrect reading on the instrument panel. No one aboard that aircraft had been in any real danger, but the pilot was not to know that, and had acted perfectly correctly in the circumstances. By the time Miss J. was safely in the terminal building her mind had already swung into action by deciding that flying was dangerous and had immediately erected its protective barrier.

As will be recalled from earlier comments, the main concern of the unconscious mind is our survival and while that same mind is capable of making decisions it is totally incapable of any form of logic. In the case of mental blocks, the terror of the conscious mind is what registers in the unconscious, its reaction being instantaneous. Once their blocks had been located and they were able to adjust to the situations which had caused them, Mr McK. and Miss J. were both as right as rain.

Time and again patients have shown how the suppression of memories can produce negative influences on their personalities. Two more adults who came to me hoping to eliminate their fear of flying were Alison P., who was an office manager and Ian L., a dental nurse. In each of these cases the fear was actually of *heights* rather than flying as such. But then it often is.

Alison's block dated back to the age of five when she was to be found with a male cousin of the same age scaling the high wall of a remote farm outhouse. Alison, being something of a tomboy, spent much of her time with her cousin.

On this occasion the structure up which they had climbed collapsed soon after they had stepped off it and on to the roof. The cousin looked at the ground far below and immediately fell off. Alison was rooted to the spot with fear. The barn was so remote that her cries for help were not heard for a long time. Meanwhile, the child's terror increased with every passing minute.

Ian's trouble was pin-pointed to the age of nine. Like Alison, he too was trapped, only in his case it was not on the roof of a barn, but half-way up a quarry when there seemed no escape either up or down. It was not until some years later that the fear of heights, which originated in the quarry, manifested itself. Ian and his schoolfriends had boarded the holiday jet during the hours of darkness. Curtains were drawn across the portholes but, as daylight flooded into the cabin, his classmates and teachers opened the curtains to admire the seascape below.

Ian also opened his curtains, took one look and panicked. He promised himself that this, his first flight, would be his last. He had heard the captain's announcements that they were flying at so many thousand feet, that they were now crossing the Atlantic and would soon be landing at New York, but the reality of being up so high in the sky had not hit him until now. Somehow, he managed to survive the holiday and the homeward journey, but he had never ventured on another flight.

Alison and Ian, having faced up to their fear by means of regressive therapy, each realized its cause and accepted it for what it was.

Being physically sick

Here is an extract from a letter received from Miss S.L. of London: 'I have just finished reading *The Power of the Mind* and wonder if you can help me. For as long as I can remember I have had a fear of being sick, or of people being sick anywhere near me. It would be lovely to be able to walk out of the front door and put this fear behind me. I am twenty-five years old.'

Miss S.L. had a professional career and was managing to control her fear as far as she could but for obvious reasons her social life was at an all-time low. Visits to pubs, clubs, parties and general merrymaking were completely off the agenda. Business lunches and informal gatherings connected with her work were also an impossibility.

For a young woman in her twenties it was not much fun. Outside the office there was very little quality to her life. Likewise Timothy F., who was sixteen, should have been having a whale of a time with his friends; instead of which he was staying in, night after night, worrying about what he described as his vomit phobia.

In therapy, Miss S.L.'s block was attributed to the fact that her father had been a publican, his establishment being rather rough and noisy. The child's bedroom was located directly above the exit into the back yard. A sensitive little thing, her system could never become accustomed to the antics of the inebriated regulars below, particularly when excessive consumption of alcohol produced its inevitable results.

Timothy's problem originated with the illness and subsequent death of an elderly aunt, who had had stomach problems for as long as anyone in the family could remember.

To add to the youth's predicament, Tara, his girlfriend, was now suffering from bulimia nervosa (the condition in which sufferers go on eating binges, then compensate by making themselves sick). Nothing, he said, would induce Tara to seek help for her illness for the simple reason that the girl did not believe herself to be ill. That was a shame, because half Timothy's problem was Tara. While regressive hypnotherapy succeeded in completely removing Miss S.L.'s phobia (she had long since moved away from the environment which had activated it), the technique could only partially help Timothy. The best I could do for the teenager was teach him to relax and to use his self-hypnosis to counteract the effects of Tara's behaviour.

As he was about to leave my young patient had a thought: 'Should I try and persuade Tara to come and see you?' he asked.

'I wish I could say yes, Timothy, but I'm afraid the answer has to be no. As you said yourself, Tara doesn't believe she has any form of illness; until she does, there is nothing I can do. Without her co-operation, it would be pointless.'

'But if she ever decides to give it a try. . . ?'

'Then I'll be happy to see her,' I assured him.

Multiple phobias

And so to those multiple phobias referred to at the beginning of this chapter: specifically to Roz, who came to me with her friend, Penny. Roz, it will be recalled, had a pathological fear of lifts and alongside her fear was serious, long-term depression. Well, hers proved a very complex case, indeed.

To begin with, it took some considerable time for Roz to relax sufficiently even to enter hypnosis, for one fundamental reason. As I had explained to Timothy, trust is absolutely essential for successful hypnotic induction and Roz found it difficult to trust anyone, least of all a stranger. I could sympathize with her predicament, but I also knew that she *really* needed help and Penny knew it too.

Because of Roz's desperate need, I persisted with her longer than I normally do and at length she began to thaw. Once she realized I was a friend and adviser and that I was not going to make a fool of her she give her implicit trust. At last we had a chance.

This patient's phobia was a bad one because it was made up of so many apparently unrelated blocks. Each had to be removed individually before we could even attempt to attack the real root of the problem. Psychological 'onion-peeling' can be a tedious and tearful process. Layer by layer must be painstakingly removed, every single block must be faced up to and disposed of, hence the need for full trust and co-operation.

'Now, Roz . . . I want you to relax. . . .' I told her. 'Deeper and deeper. . . .'

My attention was suddenly caught by the sight of Penny sitting opposite, who had tuned in to the induction and was also beginning to drift into hypnosis. It is not unusual for this to happen. Aware of the benefits, Penny's mind had decided she too could take advantage. Focusing briefly on Penny, I told her subconscious mind that I would teach her the technique of self-hypnosis later – purely for the purpose of relaxation – but that my first priority was Roz.

To Roz, who was still under hypnosis, though not yet regressed, I suggested she should ignore any instructions about to be given to Penny, and stay in her relaxed state for a few more minutes.

'Five, four, three, two, one, wide awake, Penny . . . wide awake.'

Penny opened her eyes, stretched and was fully conscious again. Now she would stay alert until I was ready to give her my full attention.

The most recent block in Roz's mind related to the breakdown of her marriage. At this stage her fear of lifts appeared symbolic. It represented her entrapment in a situation from which there seemed no escape, but there was more to her phobia than that because long after the marriage had reached its inevitable end Roz continued to suffer spasmodic attacks of depression.

This made no sense to her; she reasoned that, having put the past firmly behind her, she should be happy. She painted in something of the background to her ill-fated marriage.

A mutual love of music had brought her husband and herself together, but when the novelty had worn off they found they were totally out of tune with each other. Rather than admit defeat, Roz had put on a brave face, faked orgasms and ended up with three delightful children. But as the marriage soured the pretence faded and the effort of keeping up a front sapped her strength. The atmosphere within the household became malevolent and destructive; like many couples in their position, Roz and her husband foolishly stayed together for the sake of the children.

Eventually her man turned nasty and began proceedings for what turned out to be a particularly acrimonious divorce. In the wake of her collapsed marriage the fears and phobias – which had always been lurking in the background – began to attack with a vengeance. Her confidence vanished; her self-esteem hit an all-time low.

Chasing away the monsters in this woman's mind was no easy task. While she *had* consciously remembered her marriage before being regressed, her UNS had shielded her from the worst of it, and also from the accompanying emotions. As the full set of related memories gushed back into her mind she recalled all sorts of unsavoury aspects previously blocked off. Penny's presence helped considerably as Roz re-experienced her ordeal. She saturated her own pocket handkerchief then worked her tearful way through the box of tissues I keep on hand for precisely this type of situation.

It was time to call a halt and leave any more mental exploration for another occasion. Having taught Roz to relax, I made her promise she would practise self-hypnosis daily.

When she felt ready to have a further attempt at regression, she could let me know and we would fix a further appointment, again, preferably in the company of her friend. '. . . and the box of tissues,' she quipped.

Six weeks later a tentative telephone call from Roz told me she was ready to try again. Since seeing me she had felt better, she said.

Depression still hit her from time to time, but she managed to keep it at bay by means of self-hypnosis.

'And how do you feel about lifts now?' I asked.

'I'm afraid they still give me the creeps.'

'That's because your block has only been partially removed. Once we've cleared your memory completely you won't be frightened of them any more.'

'Is that a promise?'

'It's a promise.'

Meanwhile there was something else she could do. If she found herself faced with a situation likely to cause panic and there was no time to put herself into a state of self-hypnosis, she could give her mind a short, sharp order by saying:

'At the count of five you, my own unconscious mind, will stop this panic. That is an *order*.' By the time she had counted to five, her UNS would have responded. The appointment was fixed for two days hence. She would, she told me, be accompanied by Penny as requested.

Roz arrived early for her next appointment. She had been practising self-hypnosis several times a day and found it very relaxing.

She had also on two separate occasions felt the need to use the emergency 'count-to-five' instruction and to her amazement *that* had worked, too. Roz looked and sounded much better. For one thing, the despondency had gone; for another, she actually smiled occasionally. It was good to see her like that, but we still had some way to go. This time she responded readily and with the marriage-related block out of the way an attempt was made to direct her memories back to her days as a single woman. We had a clear run for a few years until we arrived at her senior schooldays: another unhappy period of Roz's life.

To cut what proved to be a very long story short, it was necessary to remove several blocks caused by the remarks of insensitive teachers, a house-move just as she was about to take A levels, fear of failing her exams and worry about possible career choices. With those out of the way and the fast rewind button of her mind pressed once more we were able to proceed a stage further, but instead of speeding past her junior school days the memory tape came to an abrupt halt again at the age of seven. As on the previous occasion I felt it was time to leave any more attempts at regression for another time.

In all Roz came to visit me three times over a period of several weeks before we reached the deepest and most traumatic of all her hidden memories. Copious tears accompanied the recall as the then timid, bespectacled child succumbed to repetitive bullying from her classmates, her unhappiness compounded by a series of silly little episodes in childhood which would make no sense to anyone other than a nervous, sensitive little girl.

It is understandable for a child to be upset over some trivial incident (or series of them), but it is not necessary for the adult to suffer in the aftermath. Regressive hypnotherapy enables the patient to see the situation in a new light. It also provides the therapist with some astonishing insights; although I must make a general point about patients being regressed to childhood.

If, in a state of unconscious recall, a patient uses the past tense, then something is blocking the memory and preventing true regression. In other words, the conscious mind is interfering. If those being regressed, directed back to the age of, say, three months, start describing the environment to which they have been regressed, something is radically wrong with that regression.

How many small babies are capable of verbal communication? In a true regression, the patient would once again be unable to speak. Roz did not slip up here. During all of her therapeutic regressions, she spoke in the present tense and adopted the appropriate voice-changes and mannerisms as she relived (rather than simply remembered) each episode. With each of her later blocks removed, Roz regressed easily to the age of six; at which point her reactions were such that I recognized very deep hurt.

Whatever had traumatized her then must have caused major upset in her young life. Under no circumstances would I have put her through any more block-removal that day; returning her memories to the present I gave her a booster dose of relaxation therapy. At what was to prove to be the last of Roz's visits we tackled her final block. It was, as I had suspected, caused by an incident which would have had a major psychological impact in the life of any child: namely the death of her mother.

The circumstances surrounding that death were at the root of all Roz's problems, as I was to discover. What transpired was that the unfortunate woman had been suffering from some long-term debilitating illness for which, at that time, the only available treatment was bed-rest and fresh air. This meant a period in hospital, and Roz's mother's ward was on the airy top floor of the building. With open visiting allowed, Roz and her father spent as much time as possible with the sick woman; this meant daily, sometimes twice daily, visits to the bedside over a period of many months. On arrival at the hospital they always used the lift. This meant that in the mind of the little girl lift travel became associated with sickness and death. Here, at last, we had the true cause of Roz's amnesia.

Here, way back in early childhood, was where her unconscious mind had set the wheels of its protective mechanism in action. At the risk of repeating myself let me emphasize yet again the power of the unconscious mind: the ability to store away all our experiences and actions in its internal computer. The case of Roz – and all those other patients in need of regressive hypnotherapy – clearly demonstrates the point.

To access the rich, hitherto unknown, material stored away so carefully and to extract the relevant data one must first tap into the computer and find the right program. Only by plugging into these deeply etched circuits can we determine what is happening in the innermost layers of the human mind.

Roz's memories were now crystal clear. Theoretically she should have been fine, but there was still a worry niggling away at the back of her mind.

It was an innate fear that she might have inherited her mother's disorder and that her depressions were also hereditary. The situation called for some straight talking, and I spoke with some authority: 'Now listen to me, Roz. You told me when you first came that your doctor said there was nothing physically wrong with you. Right?'

'Right,' she confirmed.

'If you doubt his diagnosis and *believe* yourself to be suffering from any form of illness, that belief could prove strong enough to bring it on. Worrying about your health is not only pointless, but dangerous.'

She got the message and left the clinic in a happier and more positive frame of mind. On the telephone a few days later, I hardly recognized her voice because she sounded so pleased with herself.

'I stepped inside a lift the day after I saw you and there wasn't a trace of panic,' she enthused. 'I zoomed up to the fourth floor of a block of flats, then down again, no problem. Since then I've been using lifts in multi-storey car parks, shopping precincts, department stores. Everywhere. I don't feel in the slightest bit depressed any more. I feel great: like I could go shooting up the Eiffel Tower, or the Empire State Building.

'Thank you *so* much for your help.

Nearly a year on, word has just reached me that Roz has found a new partner, her children are delighted with the choice and, for the first time in her life, she is truly happy. I wish her well.

Our childhood memories are not always what they seem. Some, instead of being true, personal recollections of specific episodes in our life, are snippets of information inserted afterwards by parents or relatives. In such cases the patient cannot possibly relive an event never experienced in the first place, which brings us back to the fundamental difference between remembering and reliving. With the first, patients see again the events as if watching a film or a series of photographs; with the second, they experience again all the accompanying fear and emotion.

With Roz's regression to childhood, I mentioned that when reliving early memories people must communicate in the appropriate manner. Those who continue, in order to regress to babyhood and birth itself, obviously cannot communicate at all, but will have been instructed to retain the memories and provide the details upon arousal, which they then proceed to do.

There have been occasions on which patients' mental blocks have been formed by breech deliveries, the tightening of the umbilical cord around the neck, or the pressure of forceps on the face. Having been regressed safely through their life with no mental barrier yet located, these patients are able to relive every moment in great detail and (having been instructed to bring back all the memories) to recall their experiences with crystal clarity in order to dispose of the whatever it was that caused their phobias.

In passing, I might mention that those who have been given the ability to remember their time in the womb report to having had foetal memories of warmth, comfort, swishing sounds – presumably of the amniotic fluid – and a loud banging sound which, one might assume, would represent the mother's heartbeat. The act of being born brings back memories of pressing, pushing, in some cases of the strangulation by the cord, in others of the head being manipulated and then sudden brightness as they emerge into the world. Some, having adopted a foetal position, jerk spasmodically, then give a loud, eerie scream in the manner of a new-born infant. They do not speak while re-experiencing birth, because they could not speak at the time; the descriptions, as with all these very early memories, come later.

It would appear, therefore, that some experiences in uterine life do bear a direct relationship to various mental states arising in adulthood. It is intriguing to examine mental barriers rooted in events which apparently occurred during or before birth; but barriers of this kind occur so infrequently that I do not propose to dwell on them here.

PART FIVE

When Hypnotherapy Cannot Help

13   Unwilling, or Unable

Misconceptions

One reason why hypnosis remains in the realms of the unorthodox
could be because the instrument of observation is the same as that
which is observed – the human mind. Those who feel they do not
wish to be dependent upon another person speak of the importance of retaining their individuality. This is nonsense; there is no
question of one person 'imposing his will' on another. Time and
again I find myself having to explain that all the therapist does is
open the door separating conscious and unconscious minds. I
simply teach people how to use an extra part of their own brain;
whether they choose to avail themselves of the ability is entirely up
to them.

Fear and lack of understanding will stop people going under
hypnosis; some only reach the initial stages, then for one reason or
another refuse to co-operate further. Others simply cannot grasp
the concept of what hypnosis is, or how it works. They are generally unaware of the role it can play in terms of health.

Questions are sometimes raised about safety: whether those
under hypnosis would remain in their apparent 'sleep' state if, for
example, fire were to break out around them. The answer to that
one is that, like sleep, self-hypnosis has its own safeguards.

The impact of traffic noise barely disrupts the sleep of people
who live on main roads and are constantly exposed to heavy vehicles rumbling past their window; once the unconscious mind
decides that the sounds pose no threat, it no longer disturbs the
sleepers, but if their door handle clicks they immediately awaken.

Take the case of a husband and wife, fast asleep in their bed, when suddenly in the middle of the night the baby cries.

The cry penetrates the depths of both parents' unconscious, but the reaction to it differs. The mother's UNS listens to the call and responds by waking her up immediately to check on the child's welfare. The father's UNS also listens, and also responds, but instead of alerting him to wakefulness it emits a message to his sleeping mind that the mother will attend. Obviously, if the mother is unable to do so the father's UNS will spring into action and *he* will be the one to see to the crying baby.

Just as when we are driving a car, if the conscious starts wandering and we begin to think of issues other than the road ahead, the unconscious (our internal watchdog) takes over to protect us. It is a dab hand at making decisions for us without even asking. That is why the mother, undisturbed by routine nocturnal sounds, will always be aroused by the cry of her baby. It is why, at the first hint of danger – real or imagined – the hypnotized person will immediately become fully alert.

Once I have taught patients self-hypnosis and they are back in their waking state, I always conduct a little test to satisfy myself that they have got the message.

To determine the full extent of control they now have over their unconscious, I ask them – for a few seconds and with no help from me – to lock their eyes or their hands tightly together, or to immobilize their vocal chords until they say, or even think, the word 'cancel'. When their UNS has responded to that self-instruction, everything is back to normal.

Patients sometimes remark that they could have *forced* open their eyes or hands, or *made* themselves speak. They have missed the point. *Of course* they could have done either, but their action would have destroyed the therapy. They themselves know whether their eyes or hands are locked, whether their voice is suddenly silenced.

Not for Harry
Thanks to the many misconceptions surrounding the technique, some people will simply not avail themselves of hypnosis under any

circumstances. Harry S. was one such, but his wife Evelyn did not know this when she approached me on his behalf.

Her request was straight and to the point:

'I am writing on behalf of my husband, in the hope that you might be able to help him. He suffers from multiple sclerosis and doesn't seem to be responding to conventional treatment. Harry doesn't know I am writing to you. I want it to be a surprise.

'I thought if you could fit him in for an appointment, I could just bring him along and see how we went from there. It would be wonderful if he could be cured. What do you think? Could you help him at all? If not, there's nothing lost.

'Harry won't know anything about it, because the address and telephone number on this letter are my friend's. If you write, she'll pass on your letter. If you ring, she'll take a message. Please tell me what you think.'

Evelyn's letter is reproduced verbatim because of the many points it raises. First of all, she wants to surprise her husband. Now, while the idea of arranging a surprise appointment might sound exciting to Evelyn, it is not practicable, because the patient's trust and co-operation are crucial right from the start.

Next, she remarks on how wonderful it would be if he could be cured. Evelyn's use of the word 'cure' is inappropriate because, as I emphasized to her, make clear to all those with whom I come in contact, and have reiterated throughout the pages of this book, I do not *cure* anyone.

I teach patients self-hypnosis as a possible catalyst towards self-cure. Practised regularly in the manner taught, self-hypnosis can be shown to slow down the progress of various degenerative diseases (of which MS is one) and help the patient tolerate any prescribed medications, but the process does need to be instigated by the patient.

The third question raised by my correspondent is whether I can help her man. At that stage neither of us knew how Evelyn's husband might react. The only way to answer the question would be by meeting him face to face and testing his response to the induction. While I would be perfectly happy to make an appointment for Harry, the request must come direct from him. With the best will in the world, it is no good trying to coerce someone into trying this form of treatment.

Admirable though Evelyn's intentions were, they were misguided. I had no option but to tell her so. All too often, when the approach is made by other members of the family, it is because they think hypnosis will benefit the person concerned, but that person may not necessarily agree, may not wish to be treated. As with Evelyn's Harry, they may not even be aware that such a request has been made on their behalf.

I had yet to discover whether Evelyn's husband was in favour of attempting hypnotherapy. Even if he was, so much would depend on motivation and the strength of his desire to be helped. As it happened, he was not. A tearful Evelyn telephoned to say that, having spoken to Harry, she was appalled to discover that he equated hypnosis with spells, mumbo-jumbo, swinging watches, and the inevitable 'loss of will power'. The subject of 'will power' and its 'loss' crops up as often as the proverbial bad penny.

'Too strong-willed'

Philip was a twenty-eight year old salesman who claimed to be despondent over a broken romance, although 'despondent' was the last word I would have used to describe him.

The picture of success and contentment, he said he thought hypnosis might help him recover and put him in the right frame of mind for embarking on a fresh relationship. In passing, he added that he had various other problems, but failed to specify what they were. When he appeared to be under hypnosis I checked it out, as is my custom, by testing the post-hypnotic response:

'When you open your eyes, you'll feel so happy you'll want to laugh out loud,' I instructed him.

Philip opened his eyes, but did not laugh out loud, or even quietly to himself.

'Well. . . ?' I queried. 'Don't you feel any different?'

'No,' he responded, with a smug grin. 'Try again.'

Philip thought he was challenging me, but it was himself – his own unconscious mind — that he was challenging. He was the loser, not I, and I told him so.

'Oh, so you're not going to give it another try? But I'm sure you'd manage it this time,' he went on. 'It's just that I have very strong will power and don't submit easily.'

Sorry, Philip, but as far as I was concerned the consultation ended there. To proceed further with that sort of attitude would be wasting my time and his money.

Area of least success

Perhaps the most widely publicized aspect of hypnosis is its use in the field of anti-smoking therapy, yet as far as I am concerned that is the area of least success. In my experience, many people who think they want to give up cigarettes do not, they are merely passing over the responsibility to someone else. Just as patients often expect pills from their doctor to cure them despite anything they may feel or do, so they expect the hypnotist to offer a kind of invisible mental medicine to cure what they do not really want cured. I rarely take on patients making this request and when I do, it is only because of some underlying health problem for which a doctor might have referred them. And even then, the outcome is predictable.

George was a little mouse of a man who visited me in the company of his overbearing wife Rachel, who did all the talking.

'He wants to give up smoking,' she announced in the tone of a headmistress reprimanding a naughty child. George nodded silently.

'Do I take that as a yes?' I asked.

'That's right,' he assured me. 'I do.'

My custom in this sort of situation is to put the patient under hypnosis and repeat the question, this time directing it to the unconscious. George's unconscious responded that he had no desire whatever to stop smoking.

'Then why are you here?'

'Because my wife says it's a filthy habit.'

'Do you enjoy your cigarettes?'

'Yes.'

There was no point in going on with George. His wife might have wanted him to give up smoking, but his unconscious mind had given me the true answer: George himself did *not*. No one can make a smoker give up the habit but those who are sincere in their wish to do so can certainly be helped. If they learn to control their unconscious (through self-hypnosis), they can stop by themselves.

The technique of making chocolate, or cigarettes, or whatever the patient is trying to give up, seem unpleasant is called 'confusing (or disturbing) hypnosis'. In such cases the post-hypnotic suggestion must be regularly reinforced, therefore it is not advisable for controlling behaviour.

Telling people under hypnosis that in their waking state they will no longer wish to eat chocolates or smoke, that the chocolate or cigarette will nauseate them will have very little effect unless those people really want to give up their habit. The stronger the desire, the more effective the treatment; the weaker the desire, the less the effect.

I can only help people do what they really *want* to: for example, most grossly overweight people do have a basic desire to slim, although some are not prepared to sacrifice their chocolate. As a general rule hypnosis is more effective for slimmers than for smokers.

Aversion therapy provides no long term answers; indeed, a dramatic stopping of lifelong practices could result in a shock to the system which might ultimately prove less therapeutic than the continued practice of overeating or smoking. Added to the psychological problem is the very real possibility in some instances of clinical withdrawal symptoms.

Depth therapy, which involves probing the root cause of the problem, is obviously more satisfactory in terms of results whatever the nature of the problem.

Content in his wheelchair

Les F. was referred from his family doctor. Paralyzed from the waist down, he spent his days in a wheelchair, though suffering from no recognizable physical or neurological disease. The condition had developed gradually over many years. Les was not in pain, nor did there appear to be any contributory environmental factors.

The man was happily married with two teenage sons and had no financial worries, being supported by his wife, a professional woman, who earned a high salary. Under hypnosis, it was discovered that Les felt safe and secure in his wheelchair. He could discipline his sons and believed that the fact of his being handicapped would prevent his wife from finding another partner. As an able-bodied individual he would have to earn a living and face his sons on equal terms. He knew that he could never match his wife's salary, so had resigned himself to being paralyzed.

Consciously, he had believed he was substantially and permanently handicapped and that he was coping well with the management of his life. As with our smoker, George, the true information only became available to him when the link had been established with the unconscious part of his mind.

Patients under hypnosis readily respond to suggestions made by the therapist (provided they agree with them) but the beneficial effects of those suggestions only remain if they are regularly reinforced by the patients themselves. No one will accept suggestions under hypnosis which do not meet with their full approval. When this was pointed out to him, Les was faced with an agonizing choice. He believed that to have his mobility restored could result in a broken marriage, delinquent sons and a drop in his standard of living: to leave well alone meant comfort and security. Seeing no reason why he should alter his present circumstances, Les made his choice. He did not wish to receive any treatment. His family doctor was informed of the situation, his wife was not, and his case sheet was closed.

Defiant youth (Adam)

With Les I was able to determine the cause of his problem; with Adam I was not. A tall, gangly youth of sixteen, he arrived at the clinic with his parents, sat down and sprawled across the chair. There was a defiant, stubborn look about him and I was not in the least surprised to learn that he had disrupted the household with his abusive, resentful behaviour and that he was wearing his parents out. Adam was the picture of surly defensiveness; his parents were at their wits' end.

'It's not really his fault,' explained his mother, 'He's got in with the wrong crowd, haven't you, darling? He used to be such a good boy, didn't you, love. . .' Her words trailed away.

'And so happy,' explained the father, equally eager to defend his son's reputation. 'These days, all we get are long, sullen silences. Couldn't you put it into his mind to break with his gang? Then we might get somewhere.'

Sensing an uneasy relationship between these three, I turned to the object of his parents' concern:

'Well, Adam? What do you think?'

The youth shrugged his shoulders and muttered something that sounded like 'dunno'.

'Would you like to try hypnosis?' I ventured.

'Dunno,' he repeated.

His monosyllabic replies were getting us nowhere. It would have been pointless attempting to induct this character into hypnosis, for the simple reason that he was so totally unco-operative. Nor was there any trust, essential for anyone attempting hypnosis. It occurred to me that the parents' overprotection of their boy was a fundamental part of his problem and theirs. Indeed, if anyone needed help they did and I would be ready to give it to them anytime they might request it. Self-treatment could enable them to cope with their wayward son and to dispel the depression associated with his present behaviour.

Preconceived ideas

Other types of patient who will never succeed in entering hypnosis are those who come along with their own preconceived ideas of what the therapy is about. Their proud boast is that they have tried various other forms of treatment, without success. Some have even been on stress-management courses in their attempts to cope with daily pressures. They have dabbled in yoga, guided relaxation, breathing techniques, self-massage, visualization, meditation and all sorts of tension-relieving exercises. They have even taken courses in assertiveness, self-appraisal and other such skills. To no avail. What these enthusiasts fail to realize is that they are trying to cure their problems consciously instead of learning how to shut down the conscious so that they can draw on the huge range of abilities on offer from the unconscious. Healing by means of deep self-hypnosis goes far beyond anything which can be achieved with the conscious as has been demonstrated time and again.

Seeking emotional dependency

Mrs V. came to my attention when I was addressing a women's group in a neighbouring town. She had a nervous tic in her eye: a constant, involuntary twitching which had been responsible for visits to numerous therapists, orthodox and otherwise.

She had been referred to various medical experts and they, having found no physiological cause for the twitching, suggested she try complementry therapy.

'They said it was all in my mind,' she told me. 'How dare they suggest I'm imagining it. Post-menopausal problems, indeed. Outrageous it is, from so-called professionals.'

Mrs V. explained that her latest consultations had been with practitioners of selected forms of oriental healing; one of those therapists had charged her a cool £500 for a session lasting all of twenty minutes. 'And I've had a herbalist's invoice in the post this morning for another two hundred.' The statement sounded suspiciously like a boast.

She wondered if she could give hypnotherapy a try. I explained about self-treatment and she enquired about my fee. On discovering it to be a fraction of the cost of what she had been charged elsewhere, she retorted: 'Oh no. If your treatment's so inexpensive, it can't be any good.

'You see, I always go for the top of the market: fashion, footwear, jewellery, everything. And, anyway, if there's only one visit involved, it's no good to me. I need to see a therapist regularly.' I wondered why she felt this need.

I am glad we sorted the matter out there; emotional dependency is something I *never* encourage. Now some might see Mrs V. as a 'money snob'. I saw her as a sad and lonely woman, acutely in need of something to break the boredom of her life.

Admittedly, her attitude towards my fee was not one that I had previously encountered, but in other respects she was typical of many people of her age.

PART SIX

When Self-hypnosis is the Answer

14   Making it a Habit

Those who practise self-hypnosis on a daily basis emphasise its immense value. They find the treatment reduces stress and anxiety, resolves a whole host of problems and generally boosts the 'feel-good' factor. The results, spilling over into everyday life include a more relaxed, positive frame of mind and a means of coping with life, whatever problems that life might present. Self-treatment can be directly tailored to meet the health needs of each individual; as a form of self-treatment its potential is enormous.

Jim and Nuala Duxbury, Noreen Magennis
Jim Duxbury and his wife Nuala are both talented media professionals in their thirties; Noreen Magennis is Nuala's mother. Jim is a freelance press photographer, Nuala is a feature writer for women's weekly magazines. My first meeting with Jim took place in April 1996, when he was commissioned by a magazine editor to take a series of photographs to illustrate a feature about my wife's latest book.

Having completed his task Jim relaxed, and over a cup of coffee, expressed a keen interest in the type of work I was doing. He was not unfamiliar with hypnosis, having tried it for therapeutic purposes some years earlier with another therapist, but with only limited success. 'I'd always been fascinated by hypnosis,' he admitted.

He mentioned having some trouble with his right shoulder, which he attributed to his years of having had to carry around heavy cameras and bags of equipment on assignments. Recently returned from the South of France, where he had spent three years as a freelance photographer, Jim told me that he suffered from constant headaches. They occurred when he was under pressure, and, considering that he was almost permanently in that state, the headaches had become an integral part of his life. He was, he confessed, swallowing painkillers at the rate of about four a day.

Could hypnosis help him relax and gain the sort of control that would remove the pain in his shoulder and those dreadful, persistent headaches, he wondered? In passing, he mentioned that he suffered from hay-fever every spring.

I pointed out to Jim that his problems were all stress-related and once he had gained the ability to rid himself of one, all the others would automatically cease to bother him. Thus enthused, he entered hypnosis easily and learned the technique of self-hypnosis without difficulty. I gave him the customary set of pre-programmed cards to facilitate future attempts at self-hypnosis. It was good to hear that, following his one brief session with me, his health had improved considerably.

'Since I began to practise self-hypnosis every day, the headaches have all gone, and I haven't had any hay-fever, either,' he said. 'If I do feel the beginnings of a niggly pain coming on, I tell myself to remove it. I haven't had to take a single painkiller since learning self-hypnosis. I use the technique widely.

'I accidentally bit my tongue the other day and it bled quite a lot until I remembered to tell my unconscious mind to stop the bleeding and it did.

'Another area where I find it most useful is for my work. If I have a tedious job to do, I tell myself I'll enjoy it and take really good pictures.

'It never fails. It's just wonderful to have that sort of control over your own mind.'

On that first meeting with Jim he had mentioned that Nuala too was showing signs of stress, that she was suffering from recurrent headaches and was permanently tired and lethargic.

But, unusually for a highly skilled and successful journalist, she also suffered from a lack of self-confidence. Could I help her too, he wondered? And how about his mother-in-law, who had various problems, the main one being arthritis?

'Bring them along,' I suggested. 'Provided they themselves want to try hypnosis, there shouldn't be any problem.'

Nuala and Noreen, having seen the improved state of Jim's health as a result of having been taught self-hypnosis, were only too willing to have a try. So Jim brought Nuala to see me the following week and Nuala brought her mother soon afterwards. Nuala reflected on what she saw as her main problem at the time.

'All my work is done to commission; so it's not as if I had to worry about having articles accepted, yet whenever I sit down to write a feature I'd be reluctant to start. I'd feel as if a particularly unpleasant task lay ahead of me – like school homework – yet, once I'd started, I was fine.'

Nuala confessed that her first visit to me had been motivated by basic journalistic curiosity.

'Your work sounded so interesting, I wanted to try it for myself and hoped that if I succeeded in going under hypnosis it might do me some good.'

With hindsight, I confess that that had been my hope, too, because if anyone needed treatment, it was this journalist. Nuala's stress level was as high as, if not higher than, Jim's had been before treatment. The nature of her problem did surprise me, because she appeared to be making such a success of her life. Yet it was blatantly obvious that fear of failure was causing her problems, and the fear was causing depression.

She also confirmed Jim's comment about her headaches and mentioned that several other parts of her body also gave her problems. Seldom free of pain, she was dosing herself with aspirins to try and gain some relief. The stress of it all was wearing her out. She was so tired and lethargic she needed a daily nap which for a young woman of her age was unusual.

Now, having seen how easily Jim could put himself into hypnosis, she was determined to have the same ability. Nuala's confidence did need a boost, she agreed. And yes, she did need to lift the depression. While she certainly entered a deep enough state to be given access to her unconscious mind, attempts at regression to the cause of the trouble were unsuccessful because Nuala had several points where her memory was blocked. She proved to be one of those patients who fell into the 'onion-peeling' category, referred to in an earlier chapter. In other words, the mental probing *could* be done, but it would take much more time than was available that day.

I did hit one block, where – still deep in hypnosis – she appeared to be writing something. Or, to be more precise, stumbling over *attempts* to write something. It was not very clear and Nuala herself could not see where she was or what was happening. Her memories stalled and would regress no further.

Earlier in this book, I pointed out that the fastest and most successful way of alleviating depression is to relive the incident which caused it. The act of facing up to it from a different perspective dispels it.

If that is not possible, then the alternative treatment is for sufferers to instruct their unconscious mind to send away the depression or whatever happens to be causing the trouble. Those who succeed in doing this on a regular basis tell me the feeling gradually recedes further and further into the distance until it ceases to be a problem at all. It is a method which Nuala has found eminently successful.

'Even though I didn't manage to regress, I can now cope with the pressure. And if I do ever feel a twinge of anything coming on, I tell my subconscious to get rid of the feeling. It always works.'

On the subject of her depression, or reluctance to begin work, Nuala agreed that it could well be related to her fear of failure. Her father had been a pharmacist and had nurtured an ambition for one of his children to take over the business when the time came. But when she had to drop chemistry after her mock O levels, Nuala did feel a failure (despite later passing eight O levels and three A levels). Looking back, she realizes she did feel she had let her father down and she *did* fear failure.

'I now realized my health problems were all psychosomatic. Once I'd sorted them out it gave me a whole new lease of life.

'The remarkable thing is that neither of us has taken a single painkiller since being taught self-hypnosis, and we both practise it every day. I haven't had a single headache since. That awful tiredness has gone. I have far more energy.

'I use my self-hypnosis in all sorts of situations; but mainly for self-confidence.

'But something quite dramatic happened recently. For years, I'd had a little mole on my face, just to the side of my right eye. It didn't bother me much, other than being itchy from time to time, so I told my unconscious to make it go. I forgot all about it for a while, and when I remembered I glanced in the mirror and was amazed to find that it wasn't there any more. There wasn't a trace of it left.'

Noreen came to see me with debilitating arthritic pains and also agreed her self-confidence was at a low ebb. Her response to the hypnotic induction was as good as that of her daughter and son-in-law. Once she was in deeply enough for treatment I gave her the usual ability for self-treatment and she too has been using it as part of her daily life.

'It's lovely to be able to relax. I always tell myself now that when I wake up I'll be full of confidence and happy. Everyone who knows me says I'm like a different person. I still have the occasional aches and pains, but I talk to my unconscious and it makes them go. Having that sort of access is wonderful. I have some fascinating conversations with my unconscious, and the nice thing about it is that it always does what I tell it.

'It gives me a terrific advantage over others who don't have the ability.'

The pain of Noreen's arthritis never seemed to go. She admitted that before learning self-hypnosis the arthritis had produced a feeling of helplessness.

'It's wonderful to be able to ease the pain that had been affecting virtually every joint of my body. The feeling of helplessness has gone and I feel totally rejuvenated.'

Michael and Oeda O'Hara

Michael O'Hara is Managing Director, European Operations, of a large US computer software company. His office is based in the City of London. At thirty-five years old, Michael is clearly in the fast lane.

We have known each other for several years and throughout that time he has been fully aware of my hypnosis and regression practice; but for reasons best known to himself it was April 1994 before he got around to asking me to teach him self-hypnosis. With hindsight, Michael thinks he may have been a shade cynical about the whole procedure. He therefore admits to being greatly surprised at how easily he entered hypnosis.

'I work for a highly sales-oriented company and, at the time in question, was rather stressed-out. I would arrive home in the evenings exhausted, be uncommunicative and snappy with Oeda and our (then) three children – Jasmin, four, Nils, three and Amber, who was approaching her first birthday. I also suffered from occasional headaches and nosebleeds.

'The simple technique you taught me appealed because it suited my hectic lifestyle.

'I started using it straight away and since then, however busy I am, always find time to set aside five minutes every day. I have been practising self-hypnosis regularly since that one session with you and can honestly say that it has helped me enormously.

'One of the major benefits manifested itself within a few months, when my work took me on a two-year posting to Australia with my family.

'I used your form of self-treatment to stop myself suffering from jet lag, and it worked so well that I now use it every time I board a plane. I have never suffered from jet lag since, although I have been on some very long flights, including several to Hong Kong and Japan, and recently with Oeda to Mexico for an international convention. Another benefit of self-hypnosis is in coping with executive stress.'

It came as no surprise to me therefore when Oeda, impressed with her husband's new-found skills, asked if she could learn the same relaxation methods. So, on their return from Australia, that is precisely what she did. Now it was Michael's turn to be impressed.

'Oeda is a calm, unstressed person anyway,' he reflects 'but sometimes she found it difficult to unwind. She doesn't any more. By means of self-hypnosis she can relax straight away – which is some feat in a house full of children!

'During her recent pregnancy, she stepped up her use of the technique and it made her very relaxed about the whole proce-dure. She did not worry about this pregnancy at all, the delivery went perfectly and we now have another bouncing, healthy son. Finlay arrived safe and sound on 3 August 1997.'

Self-hypnosis has proved useful on other occasions, too. In May 1997, an unnerving experience might have proved even more traumatic for this energetic young couple had they not both called upon their mental abilities to ease the strain of the situation.

Michael, who commutes daily between Kent and London (an eighty-mile round trip) by motorbike, was returning home late one evening, glad to be in the open air after a particularly long working day. A few miles from home, his journey was suddenly and dramatically interrupted when a motor vehicle zoomed out from a side road. The resultant impact threw him along the road. 'I felt myself bounce a few times before coming to rest in the opposite carriageway. Fortunately – and most unusually – there was no traf-fic in that lane.' Thanks to a top quality crash helmet and leathers Michael escaped with nothing more serious than multiple bruises and shock. His machine was a write-off.

'My body ached all over until, after the immediate shock of the accident and hospital assessment and treatment of my condition, I remembered to use self-hypnosis. I was delighted to find that it removed the pain of the bruising straight away.

'I was back on form within forty-eight hours and felt no further pain.'

Oeda, heavily pregnant at the time, also managed to de-stress herself very quickly.

Concludes Michael: 'While I may have been a bit cynical once, I am certainly not any more.'

David and Cathy Groeger

At the very beginning of this book I quoted from an unsolicited letter sent to me in January 1997 by Cathy Groeger in which she mentioned the progress made by David and herself since both had learned and been practising self-hypnosis.

David and Cathy both work as chiropractors. A comparatively new form of treatment in the UK (though long-established in America), chiropractic is a form of therapy which involves manual treatment of joint disorders, mainly those of the spine. The word itself is of Greek origin and means 'treatment by manipulation'.

When I last heard from Cathy, David had just graduated and Cathy was in her final year of studies. Six months later I heard from Cathy again. Having sailed through her final exams she had started her chiropractic clinical year and, knowing I am always interested in the welfare of former patients, she updated me on the progress of her new husband and herself. But before quoting extracts from her most informative letter, let me paint in something of the background to our original meeting.

Cathy's initial approach to me was after she had watched a screening of the television programme *This Morning* in which I was making a guest appearance. She says she went straight out to obtain a copy of *The Power of the Mind*, the contents of which fanned the flames of her interest in hypnosis.

'That was six years ago. I came to see you as soon as possible and what you taught me then has helped me enormously. I was nineteen years old and slowly killing myself with stress, anxiety and self-doubt.

'My health at the time was not good. Although there was nothing in particular wrong with me, I believe I was brewing up something serious. My skin was always grey and I was constantly tired, so much so that during college holidays I spent many afternoons asleep. I was generally quite depressed.

'At times, my tiredness got so bad I really wanted to die . . . pretty sad for a teenager.' Cathy was indeed in a very low state of mind and body and acutely in need of treatment. 'The technique worked immediately. It was as if everything reversed. My skin changed to a healthy pink and I rarely felt tired. I was able to sleep properly for the first time in years. My head cleared, I felt that now I could influence my own state of health. Above all, I felt in control of things rather than letting myself be swept along as before.

'What you taught me changed my life. I would certainly not be doing chiropractic but for you, which means that I would not have met my husband, with whom I am very happy.' Nor, she adds, would she have performed so well at her studies. 'Since using self-hypnosis to improve my memory, I have never suffered the sort of memory blanks I used to when faced with exam papers. In fact, I used the exam hypnosis last week, having already used it for the assessments last term. The technique calmed me down, too.

'For the past three years, my exam results have been pretty good and I feel confident about them. Before knowing about self-hypnosis and putting it into practice, I was in the habit of failing. Now, on the odd occasion when I have forgotten to use it before tests, my old nerves surface and my performance suffers.'

Cathy introduced me to David shortly before their marriage in August 1996. Their visit, she says, proved 'the best thing we ever did.' David was suffering from eczema and responded as well to the treatment as had his (then) fiancée. He learned and practised self-treatment and after a few months discovered that the treatment was beginning to clear up the patches on his legs. Then, when they had almost entirely disappeared, he lapsed a little.

'Although David doesn't use his self-hypnosis very often, his eczema patches are much better and so is his general health. It is as if his system is working properly at last.' Cathy has found hypnosis such a fascinating form of therapy that she attended a short course in London (not, incidentally, run by myself) during 1996, with a view to practising it alongside the work in which she herself is now fully qualified.

'I'm still having a few misgivings as to whether chiropractic gets to the root of the problem,' she reflects, 'but that's probably because I know about hypnosis. After my brief course in it, I have begun to realize that therapeutically, it has a lot to offer. Other courses appear deficient when compared to your method, which always seems to hit the mark.'

Rob K. (*victim of a beating*)

Rob K. is a fifty-year-old man whose back was fractured in a beating many years ago. His spine healed, but the legacy of pain and arthritis on the site of the injury severely disabled him. A reformed alcoholic, Rob also suffered over a lengthy period from the effects of drinking. 'My back problem varied from a dull ache to the sort of searing pain that made me cry out in agony.

'On top of the pain and depression, I was suffering from dreadful withdrawal symptoms, was pronounced mentally ill and put on heavy medication. Instead of curing me the medication made me worse. Anyone with personal knowledge of this sort of life style will understand that recovering from drink is one thing, regaining mental sobriety is quite another.'

Rob had already won the battle over his alcoholism before I met him in 1992. It was for his back problem that he sought my help. The pain, he confessed, was so bad at times that he was sorely tempted to give in to his craving. There's nothing quite like pain and depression to weaken the resolve. 'If I go under hypnosis and it eases my backache, will it also help me keep away from drink?' he asked. 'Because, right now, I'm really beginning to struggle.'

To his credit, Rob had not had a drink for more than a year and I was only too happy to try and help him. Because he was showing such remarkable control over his conscious mind, I pointed out how much more he could do for himself with access to the unconscious.

Rob was a highly intelligent, strongly motivated man. As anticipated, he showed no resistance whatever to the hypnotic induction and was soon at the very deepest level. I taught him self-hypnosis and knew in my heart of hearts that he would grasp it with both hands. I knew too that he would never let it go. This man would use it not only for the purpose of sobriety, but for pain relief and to counteract all those nasty negative feelings associated with depression and stress.

And sure enough, after a few days he was on the telephone: 'Self-hypnosis is wonderful,' he declared. 'I've never known anything like it. I'd been finding it particularly difficult to relax when the yearning for alcohol began creeping up on me, but now

I just tell the feeling to go away, and it does. I don't know what to say.'

'Just carry on giving your unconscious the necessary instructions,' I told him. 'I'm delighted you're doing so well.'

Five years on, Rob is still managing to fight off what he calls 'the demons' inside him. Because I happen to be in his neighbourhood fairly regularly I pop in for a chat and a cup of tea when I'm around. Sometimes I give him a booster but mostly we just chat and he brings me up to date on his progress.

Alcoholics can never be 'cured', but their condition can be controlled and that control is enough for Rob. He knows he is winning. His physical problems are also on the wane. There is still an area of tenderness around his neck, and some inflammation in the region of his back, but the discomfort bears no comparison to the constant, nagging pain he had suffered for so long before embarking on self-hypnosis. In time they should go away completely. Rob concludes: 'When I'm in pain, my muscles go very tense and nothing relaxes them like self-hypnosis. It's as if heat was being generated up and down my back and round my shoulders. The way the unconscious mind responds to instructions is amazing.'

Isn't it, just!

15   Conclusion

The comparison of the human brain to a computer might be dismissed as simplistic by some people. They might argue that, although both use electrical circuits to operate, one human brain has infinitely more connections than the entire Internet system. That is, of course, true. It is also true that, with no sensory input, the computer is not a thinking machine, therefore the programmer must be careful to input accurate information, in order for the machine's output also to be accurate.

When incorrect programs are stored in a computer incorrect messages are transmitted. The errors must be corrected or those wrong messages will continue to beam out, causing chaos in a variety of damaging ways, with the ultimate possibility of network failure in the computer, or varying degrees of health problems – from mild to totally devastating – in the human.

Correct the faulty program in either and a satisfactory result will be achieved. Once the correct process has been activated we, like the computer, have the ability to recall anything stored in the memory bank. I therefore consider the comparison to be valid.

Genetic diseases like cancer, arthritis and certain heart conditions arise because of faults in the genetic code and inherited gene faults can put us at risk of disease. The trouble with cancer is that it is not one condition, but several. Cancer results from cells running riot; the way to treat those cells is to correct their riotous route, isolate, or destroy them. Cells, on becoming malignant, multiply in places where they can damage and destroy healthy tissue.

When inducting people into hypnosis, the reason that I instruct antigens to combine with antibodies is because the combination restores cells to normality *provided* the patient's UNS responds correctly and *provided* the bodily destruction has not already progressed beyond the point where it can be repaired.

We have seen (chapter 6), how self-hypnosis has been success-fully used to help patients suffering from various types of cancer. The aim of teaching self-hypnosis is to restore health to normal. If this cannot be achieved, then the treatment can at least be made to improve people's ability to cope with their illness or changed circumstances.

In a hospital or hospice, self-treatment of this type can be seen to ease pain, discomfort and the distress associated with adjustment to a chronic or life-threatening disease. Being able to turn off pain and relax makes quite a difference to a patient's quality of life and sense of well-being.

Helping patients into a relaxed state in a safe environment and teaching them skills they can continue to use unaided helps them cope with their illness. While high-technology aspects of medicine and nursing may be essential to sustain life, patients tell me that the ability to practise self-hypnosis every day is a bonus and makes a very great difference to their lives. An increasing number of doctors, nurses and other professionals admit that this supportive therapy has real benefits in that it helps alleviate disabling symp-toms and enables patients to tolerate prescribed medications.

Stress is a major problem in society today and it is significant that the medical profession is at last beginning to take some interest in the subject, not only in how it affects their patients but also them-selves.

When a group of psychiatrists gathered together recently a major topic for discussion came under the heading of Work and Stress in Medical Practitioners.[1] Their findings revealed that doctors, nurses, managers and professionals allied to medicine experienced higher levels of stress than the general population.

Dr Gillian Hardy, of the Psychological Therapies Research

Centre, University of Leeds, told delegates that a survey of eleven thousand employees from nineteen NHS trusts in England organized by the psychiatrists showed that women doctors and women managers had particularly high levels of stress. Their survey also revealed a curious fact: namely that depression and stress were Western phenomena.

Dr Dinesh Bhugra, of London's Institute of Psychiatry, spoke on the subject of depression.

He said that a series of focus groups carried out among Punjabi women living in London had found no Punjabi equivalent of depression, although all participants had been aware of the condition. Focus groups, he explained, were a method in social science research for obtaining knowledge of problems relating to minority ethnic groups. Apparently, the women interviewed saw depression as being related to life's stresses. Dr Bhugra added: 'They viewed depression as caused by life events like unemployment, financial difficulties, bereavement, family conflict and racial events.' Here is the interesting bit. 'They saw the treatment as essentially non-medical using alternative healers, religious priests, friends and talking therapies'.

The effects of the contrasting Western tendency towards conventional medicine and social stigma are evidenced in the case of a Scottish patient of mine whom I shall call Eileen, which is not her real name. Eileen was a skilled and talented schoolteacher in her forties. She had taught a succession of children in the junior section of her school for years when, suddenly, the deputy head-mistress was forced to take early retirement for medical reasons. Eileen was appointed as her replacement. She proved as successful an administrator as she was a teacher and her prospects were excellent. It was rumoured that, on the head teacher's retirement next year, Eileen would be her natural successor.

An attractive and elegant woman, she prided herself on her looks, particularly her luxuriant red hair. And it was the hair that brought her to my clinic: or, more precisely, the loss of it. Over a period of weeks – or was it months, she wondered? – her hair had started coming out in clumps. Not only that, there was a noticeable bald patch behind one ear. Her hairdresser had attributed it to stress and suggested that she should seek professional help. Incensed, Eileen had stormed out of the salon and taken her custom elsewhere.

Eileen had been in her post for long enough to recognize the signs of stress and knew that only incompetent teachers allowed their work to get on top of them. What right had a hairdresser to suggest she was not coping with her job?

Though loath to do so, she visited her doctor, expecting him to give her some sort of cream, or spray, to clear up what she considered to be a minor problem of some sort with her scalp. Instead, he confirmed the hairdresser's findings, diagnosed stress and referred her to me.

Regression proved what I had suspected: the date of her hair loss coincided with the date of her promotion. She worried incessantly about her ability to deal with all the paperwork, knew that she was in line for further promotion, but feared that what she perceived as her own incompetence would result instead in demotion. On top of all her new responsibilities was the event she dreaded most: the school inspector's visit. She was thoroughly ashamed of herself for being so stressed. Such a state of mind was hardly the mark of a good teacher, she stated.

I had to agree, but told her that if she learned the technique of self-hypnosis and practised it on a daily basis, she would no longer suffer from the condition.

'And my hair. . . ?' she asked, almost apologetically. 'I know it sounds vain, but will my hair stop falling out?'

'If you succeed in going under hypnosis, you can control that hair loss yourself and make it grow back without any problem. More important, you can get rid of the stress which is causing the alopaecia, and stop worrying about paperwork, inspectors, demotion and everything else.'

Eileen's IQ was so high that she entered hypnosis in record time. Her response was excellent throughout and having given her the routine treatment for stress and satisfied myself that she was capable of self-hypnosis, I suggested she advise her unconscious to stop the hair loss and all those other negative feelings connected with her work, particularly her fear of demotion.

I gave her a set of my 'customized' cards and advised her to instruct her unconscious on a daily basis with whichever message was relevant to the day; be it connected with her colleagues, her paperwork, or the dreaded inspector. But she must always input two specific messages to the files of her mental computer: 'You, my unconscious mind, will make me fully confident about myself and my pupils. That is an order,' and 'You will continue regrowing my hair until all the loss has been replaced, and you will never allow me to become so stressed that my hair falls out again.'

Eileen called in to see me on her way home from school a few weeks later, to tell me how she was getting on. The stresses and strains of her job were no longer getting to her. She was coping admirably with everything. Even the inspector's visit, she quipped, had not made her turn a hair.

'Speaking of which, look. . . .' I was most gratified to see that the patch behind her ear was no longer bald. The alopaecia was gone and with it all her fears and dreads, particularly the one about being demoted. She beamed broadly. 'The Education Authority has just confirmed that I take over as head teacher next year,' she announced. 'And I have you to thank for all that.'

'No,' I corrected her. 'You have *yourself* to thank. And to congratulate. I'm delighted you're doing so well. Just make sure you don't ever let yourself get into that stressed state again.

'Meanwhile, I think you should have a little word with the hair-dresser who first picked up on your condition, and tell her she was right, after all.'

'I've already done so,' she told me. 'I'm back on her books now, anyway.'

I am sure Eileen is coping well in every aspect of her work and will continue to do so.

Throughout this book we have been looking at the brain and explaining the human body's two kinds of mind. We have seen how the greater portion (the UNS) never sleeps, not even in the setting of a hospital theatre when under the influence of a general anaesthetic.

On the few occasions when patients have regressed (at their own request) to some surgical procedure, they have repeated the overheard conversations taking place between surgeon, anaesthetist, theatre sister and other members of the team. Interspersed with the surgeon's requests for instruments and the medical jargon accompanying such a procedure, are snatches of general conversation. As reported, these invariably relate to inconsequential matters, such as which football team each supports, the repeating of dinner party gossip and talk of children's progress at school.

One patient recalled music being played, silenced during a period of crisis, and resumed when the crisis was past. The ability to hear and mentally register one's surroundings when the conscious mind has been shut down is a medically accepted fact.

That is why, when patients are in coma as Brian's wife was (chapter 7), those visiting the bedside are encouraged to speak to them. The conscious may be out of action but the unconscious never is. It is constantly listening, watching, and doing everything in its power to help us back to health. Even when all our bodily functions are winding down the UNS is still watching over us. When death is imminent and the system is about to close down permanently, hearing is the last of our senses to go. Brian's wife would have heard his repeated declarations of love and it was important for him to know that.

The complexities of the human – or, more specifically, the *unconscious* human – mind are such that it can spring into action at the oddest moments. In my earlier book[2] I referred to a woman who had single-handedly lifted a motor car right up off her young grandson whose legs had been trapped by the vehicle. A similar – if somewhat less weighty – problem occurred in our own household. A few years ago Ronnie, our large dog (Dalmatian x bull terrier crossbreed), jumped over the front gate but did not make it to the pavement because, immediately after vaulting over, his left hind paw became stuck in the wrought iron and he was incapable of freeing it. As he swung helplessly upside down, his cries sent my wife (who weighs all of eight stone) running to the gate and, having freed the paw, she lifted the injured animal high over the gate and carried him into the house to await the vet's arrival.

The dog, though young and only recently arrived in our home, settled down in a corner and lay quietly until professional help arrived. That dog is such a heavy, muscular animal that in ordinary, everyday life my wife does not have the strength to lift him off the ground. I relate this story to demonstrate two points. The first is to confirm my earlier statement about our bodies being capable of superhuman strength (probably due to the rush of adrenalin), when necessary, the second is in support of my claim that animals appear to have retained their innate ability which we, as humans, have largely lost: that is, to switch off pain until its cause can be attended to.

To return to the story of Ronnie. The paw, though badly injured and with fractures so compound it was almost beyond redemption, was surgically repaired. Thanks to skilful orthopaedic work, amputation proved unnecessary and once the broken bones were set and the shattered limb rebuilt, the dog's own healing system went into operation. Today there is no swelling, no weakness, he does not even limp. (Nor, for that matter, has he made any further attempts to jump over the gate.) Another important point is thus demonstrated: it is that animals have also retained their ability for self-healing.

When we injure ourselves two things happen. First, the area affected is damaged. This happens immediately, the pain and inflammation come later. The original stimulus-message sent from the site of the wound to the brain blocks the pain response in the animal and it should do so in us. The next message is to set the process in motion for the healing to be completed.

We too can remove the pain of a fractured limb once we know how to set the wheels in motion (painkillers have a nasty habit of hiding critical symptoms). We too can reduce swellings and restore normal functioning. If domestic animals can respond directly to internal stimuli why should the human body, with its more sensitive nervous system, not be able to do so?

As for lifting heavy weights in moments of crisis: it can be disconcerting to discover you have just done something you know is impossible, particularly if you do not understand how you managed it. The process is, like all other processes, activated deep in the unconscious.

It is not unknown for paralyzed people to walk out of their wheelchairs after their UNS has been instructed to set about restoring mobility. While the normal reaction to this phenomenon would be to ensure that the healing process continues until mobility is fully restored, some patients – when they realize what has happened – are so terrified by what they believed to have been impossible that they find their state of mind unready or unwilling to accept it. I consider it crucial, therefore, always to give patients confidence in their own ability and in calming, reassuring tones, insist that they must never doubt that the suggested improvement will be achieved.

When the foetus is in the womb, we believe it can hear because, when those under hypnosis are taken back to early recollections and their pre-birth memories are tested, the evidence seems to point in that direction, though one can only speculate on how well developed the sense of hearing is at that stage. The results of regressing grown men and women back to a time when they were in the mother's womb seems to indicate that the foetus has the ability to recall memories of swishing and pulsating.

The ability to hear is believed to develop almost as early as the ability to move (roughly around the fourth month of gestation), and although I can offer no evidence to show from these uterine memories that as well as hearing the mother's body sounds the foetus can also hear external noises through the abdominal wall, I believe it to be so. Pregnant women who sing and play music to their unborn babies do tend to produce an inherent love of music in those babies. Mind you, environment helps, too.

The children of musical parents who grow up in a musical household inevitably find some of it rubs off. Mothers who envelop themselves in an atmosphere of music when pregnant tend to pass on that love of music to their children. The mother of Phoebe, the 'cellist (chapter 7), was one such, which could account for Phoebe's own love of and skill with music. Likewise Estelle, the budding concert pianist (chapter 12), who mentioned casually that both of her parents were gifted singers.

I hope that it now becomes clear to all those who wish to try this form of therapy that there is nothing sinister or metaphysical about my work. I simply help patients view themselves in a new light and show them how to get their minds working in such a way that they can take control of themselves.

There is no doubt that self-hypnosis activates the healing process in order to bring about an improvement in the patient's general condition and that it can be a most effective means of preserving our health. Good health is the birthright of every man, woman and child who ever lived or ever will live upon this earth. Throughout this book I have attempted to show how we can rediscover long-lost abilities and sharpen them up, not just to prolong life, but to make the very best of it for as long or as short as that life may be.

Notes

1 Hardy, Dr Gillian, Stress in the NHS highest among women doctors and women managers; Bhugra, Dr Dinesh, Punjabi women found to have different concepts of depression. Two reports from The Royal College of Psychiatrists Annual Meeting, Bournemouth (England), 1–4 July 1997.
2 Keeton, Joe with Simon Petherick, *The Power of the Mind*, (Robert Hale, 1989), p.101.

Epilogue

A challenge for doctors

In 1981 I issued a challenge to the medical profession[1] and have been issuing it on a regular basis ever since, so far without any reaction. No one seems very interested in taking it up. My challenge runs something like this: bring me a group of, say, twenty-four patients suffering from migraine and/or arthritis. Make it what you yourselves call a blind trial. *You* select the patients, *you* decide on the circumstances under which we hold the meeting and *you* choose the venue. Keep the age of the patients below forty-five and I will teach twenty of them how to rid themselves of pain. With older patients, the success rate drops proportionately because the older we are, the more we resist change.

The challenge is available for the scientific board of the British Medical Association, or any other medical group interested in having evidence offered in the presence of an impartial observer. All right, so my methods may be considered by some to be non-scientific, but does that really matter? In the final analysis, the issue at stake is surely whether they work, or not.

During his stint as Senior Lecturer in International Community Health at the Liverpool School of Tropical Medicine, Dr David Stevenson sat in on many of my sessions and watched several patients being treated.

He believed I had probably saved the National Health Service quite a lot of money for the pills which patients no longer needed to take.[2] On the subject of pain, it makes sense to have any that

201

persists over a period of time investigated by a doctor to eliminate the possibility of some serious, underlying medical condition.

By the way, the challenge I issued all those years ago still holds. It is not restricted to doctors; medical students, nurses or any health care professionals are welcome to take it up.

Notes

1 Chamberlain, Melanie, 'Joe throws down the gauntlet to medical profession', *Sunday Extra* (Birmingham), 1 November 1981. pp.10–11.

2 Stevenson, David, Introduction, *New Hope Through Hypnotherapy*, by Monica O'Hara, Abacus (1989), p.vi.

Index